Case Studies in
Rehabilitation

Case Studies in
Rehabilitation

Patricia A. Ghikas, PT, GCS, MEd

Hale Hospital

Haverhill, MA

Michele Clopper, MS, OTR/L

Bay State College

Boston, MA

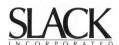

SLACK
INCORPORATED

an innovative, information, education, and management company
6900 Grove Road • Thorofare, NJ 08086

ISBN: 978-1-55642-425-0

Instructors: *Case Studies in Rehabilitation: Instructor's Manual* is also available from SLACK Incorporated. Don't miss this important companion to *Case Studies in Rehabilitation*. To obtain the Instructor's Manual, please visit http://www.efacultylounge.com.

The author, editor, and publisher cannot accept responsibility for errors or exclusions or for the outcome of the application of the material presented herein. There is no expressed or implied warranty of this book or information imparted by it.

The procedures and practices described in this book should be implemented in a manner consistent with the professional standards set for the circumstances that apply in each specific situation.

The work SLACK Incorporated publishes is peer reviewed. Prior to publication, recognized leaders in the field, educators, and clinicians provide important feedback on the concepts and content that we publish. We welcome feedback on this work.

Ghikas, Patty.
   Case studies in rehabilitation / Patty Ghikas, Michele Clopper.
      p. ; cm.
   Includes bibliographical references and index.
   ISBN 1-55642-425-6 (alk. paper)
   1. Occupational therapy--Case studies. 2. Physical therapy--Case studies. I. Clopper,
Michele. II. title.
   [DNLM: 1. Rehabilitation--Case Report. WB 320 G423c 2000]
   RM735.45 .G475 2000
   615.8'2--dc21

                                                 00-049691

Printed in the United States of America.

Published by: SLACK Incorporated
                    6900 Grove Road
                    Thorofare, NJ 08086 USA
                    Telephone: 856-848-1000
                    Fax: 856-853-5991
                    www.slackbooks.com

Contact SLACK Incorporated for more information about other books in this field or about the availability of our books from distributors outside the United States.

Last digit is print number: 10 9 8 7 6 5 4

Dedication

To all that have contributed to making this book a reality—my family, students, colleagues, and most especially those individuals who I have had the privilege to know as their physical therapist.

Patty Ghikas

To my patients who challenge my creativity to provide them with treatment that is meaningful to their life and goals. To my family who have always supported and respected my choices.

Michele Clopper

Contents

Instructors: *Case Studies in Rehabilitation: Instructor's Manual* is also available from SLACK Incorporated. Don't miss this important companion to *Case Studies in Rehabilitation*. To obtain the Instructor's Manual, please visit http://www.efacultylounge.com.

Acknowledgments

This book would not be possible without the experiences provided by our patients and students.

About the Authors

Patricia Ghikas graduated from the University of Vermont with an undergraduate degree in physical therapy in 1987. She completed a certificate of graduate study in geriatric physical therapy from the MGH Institute of Health Professions in 1997, and a Master of Education degree from the University of Massachusetts–Lowell in 2000. She received her certification as a specialist in geriatric physical therapy from the American Board of Physical Therapy Specialties in 1997. She has held clinical staff positions at New England Rehabilitation Hospital in Woburn, MA; Carleton–Willard Village in Bedford, MA; Whittier Rehabilitation Hospital Home Care in Haverhill, MA; and Lawrence General Hospital in Lawrence, MA. She has held health care management positions for Advantage Health Corporation and Advanced Rehab Systems. She has provided geriatric rehabilitation consultation services through her private practice from 1995 to 1997. In addition, she has held adjunct and full-time faculty positions in the physical therapist assistant program at Newbury College in Brookline, MA from 1994 to 1999. She has written the home study series module *Treatment of the Individual with Parkinson's Disease* as an invited author for the geriatric section of the APTA, and has been an active member of the APTA of MA since 1993, holding several offices at the district level. Currently she is the Program Director for the Wound Healing Center at Hale Hospital, Haverhill, MA.

Michele Clopper graduated from Erie Community College with an Associate degree in occupational therapy and later completed her Bachelor's degree in OT at Boston University. She went on to complete a Master of Science in rehabilitation counseling from Boston University. Initially, Michele worked for over 10 years in outpatient psychiatry for veterans affairs with a specialty in providing services for Vietnam veterans with posttraumatic stress disorder. She has presented in several international conferences regarding treatment of this population, including incarcerated veterans. She has also worked in acute rehabilitation hospitals, subacute/skilled settings, and home care. She has been on the roster of accreditation for ACOTE for OTA programs for the past 6 years and has had the opportunity to serve as an Academic Fieldwork Coordinator/Instructor at Bay State College in Boston. During her career, she has always been an active mentor and has supervised OTA and OT students. Currently, she is the Director of Occupational Therapy at Tewksbury Hospital, which is a Department of Public Health facility in Massachusetts.

Introduction

In our roles as both practitioners and as educators, we have had many opportunities to work with students as they were bridging their academic experience into the clinical arena. The majority of these students express their desire for more realistic application of the clinical reasoning process prior to their fieldwork settings. There are also those students who would benefit from additional structured learning experiences to prepare them for successful clinical work. We have scrambled, at times, to provide clinical examples from our own practice to assist in the development of well-founded clinical reasoning and practice. This book is a product of our efforts to provide learning experiences for our future practitioners and to facilitate discussion regarding the melding of the patients' desired goals and our abilities to assist them in achieving those goals.

In developing these composites, we urge the reader to view each patient as a social being with "connectedness" to others, his or her community, and environment. Each case presents that particular patient's goal to return, as a whole person, to his or her desired lifestyle. One cannot underestimate the drive of each patient to achieve his or her goals and the amount of investment to participate in a treatment plan that is tailored to meet his or her values and needs.

Significant others, including caregivers, must be integrated and educated into the treatment process, for they hold an important role that helps to determine the success of the final outcome. These individuals often bear the weight of the direct implementation of our recommendations, whether it be cueing, role changes, equipment purchases, or changes in the environment. Therefore, the goals must have them in mind.

For both our patient and his or her significant other, we must always be sensitive to his or her functioning regarding abilities to cope with the changes in the patient's functioning. With rehabilitation services being implemented soon after the medical "insult," we see patients with higher levels of acuity and, sometimes, without full appreciation of their condition or possible outcome. We must tailor our approaches and treatments to make them successful and meaningful for each patient. Part of this process involves developing strong collaborative roles with other members of the treatment team.

Cohesive treatment teams afford support and validation for the patient and his or her significant other. It is comforting and strength building to hear that various members of a treatment team are in agreement regarding one's course of treatment. For the practitioner, the collaborative relationship also provides support but, more importantly, allows the practitioner to fill the gaps of his or her area of clinical expertise. It further qualifies questions such as: Is the person going to be using a walker or a wheelchair while performing cooking activities? Is the patient going to achieve functional grasp to utilize a particular ambulation device?

This book is an effort to support the development of strong collaborative occupational and physical therapy relationships for the student. It is an extremely rewarding treatment plan that is holistic, hierarchical, and successful. In order to treat successfully, we must remember that we are a part of the whole. We are not the whole. Being a practitioner in physical or occupational therapy brings many riches; one is the strong bonds of being a team player and assisting our patients in reaching their highest level of functioning. Through sharing our areas of clinical expertise, together we develop a plan that reflects respect for our patients and each other.

To enhance our working relationship, we must share some common beliefs and language regarding the health-illness continuum. This provides a basis for a cohesive treatment plan and assists in defining the level at which a patient requires intervention and why he or she requires it. For the purposes of this book, we have selected the Nagi scheme of disability. This model offers clarity for the scheme of disablement by describing the process and progression of disease as it relates to the individual's ability to function within his or her usual roles and environment. Figure 1 represents the concepts of each area of the scheme: pathology, impairment, functional limitation, and disability (Jette, May, 1994).

Nagi refers to this active pathology as the interruption of any normal cellular process. He refers to impairment as the result of pathology, whether it is a primary or secondary impairment. An example would be a patient with Parkinson's disease who has truncal rigidity and delayed initiation (primary impairment), but is then deconditioned due to immobility (secondary impairment).

A functional limitation portrays constraints in the performance of the individual. This may include cognitive deficits, ambulation, communication, transfers, etc. The disability level includes one's daily roles and activities of daily living/performance components. These may include self-feeding, childcare, work, etc. People may share similar disabilities, but they may stem from different reference points of the model.

The reader is encouraged to keep this model or his or her preferred model in mind while utilizing these cases in order to clarify his or her view of disablement. Efforts were made to provide cases that are relevant to clinical practice for the assistant and licensed level practitioner. Please refer to the appropriate documents regarding role delineation as set forth by the national association along with your state's practice act.

In conclusion, we would like to express our appreciation to all of our patients throughout the years who have trusted us and have allowed us to be a part of their lives. Our patients have taught us ways to face challenges with dignity and with reserves of emotional strength.

Active Pathology → *Impairment* → *Functional Limitation* → *Disability*

Figure 1: The Nagi scheme of disability.

Reference

Jette AM. Physical disablement concepts for physical therapy research and practice. *Phys Ther*. 1994;74:380-386.

ORTHOPEDICS

Left Hip Fracture

Josephine Walker is a 98-year-old woman who lives in the "mother-in-law" apartment in the garage of her son's new home. There are no steps to enter the apartment and no architectural barriers once inside, with the exception of the traditional tub and shower, which Josephine has difficulty entering and exiting independently. Prior to this fall, she was independent in all basic functional activities at an ambulatory level without a device. She had a housekeeper come in to do the housework once every 2 weeks. Her son and daughter-in-law did her laundry for her.

She primarily stayed at home with the exception of Mondays and Wednesdays when she was driven by family or friends to the senior center for bingo and participation in the exercise class. She also attended church faithfully on Sunday mornings with her son, his wife, their four children, and eight grandchildren. There are six steps with a rail to enter/exit the church. There is no ramp or other entrance available. She is a retired dressmaker who prides herself on her ability to continue to sew and make all of her own clothes and gifts for her family for birthdays and Christmas.

She fell in her kitchen while making dinner one evening and sustained a left subcapital hip fracture. She was admitted to the hospital and had surgery for a cemented bipolar hip arthroplasty 1 day after her fall. She was discharged to your facility 4 days later with orders for functional retraining at partial weightbearing (PWB) status (PWB for 2 weeks, then progress to weightbearing as tolerated [WBAT]).

She presents to you in the clinic with the following findings:

1. *Significant past medical history*: Osteoporosis for 25 years, congestive heart failure (CHF), cataract in right eye, status post (s/p) appendectomy 60 years ago, and 10 uncomplicated childbirths.

2. *Medications*: Tylenol III as needed (prn) and Fosimax (Merck & Co., West Point, PA).

3. *Cognition/perception*: Within normal limits (WNL) for perception.

Cognition:

- *Alert and oriented x 3*
- *Attention: No difficulty attending to tasks during this evaluation. Some decreased attention in a distractable environment.*
- *Concentration: Within functional limits (WFL).*
- *Memory: Intact long-term memory with functional short-term and recent memory. Patient reports using lists and a calendar to "keep track of things at home."*
- *Sequencing: WNL*
- *Ability to follow directions: WNL*
- *Initiation: WNL*
- *Insight/judgment: WNL*
- *Problem solving: Good for performance of her basic functional tasks.*

4. *Sensation*: Intact throughout on gross assessment for light touch, pain, temperature, pressure, and proprioception. Her pain at rest is a 3 on a 1 to 10 scale and with mobility/range of motion (ROM) 5 on a 1 to 10 scale in the left lower extremity. Otherwise she does not currently have complaints of pain.

5. *ROM:* See Table 1-1.

6. *Strength*: See Table 1-2.

7. *Skin/edema*: Intact skin integrity with the exception of a clean and dry suture line with staples intact. Severe left distal lower extremity (LE) edema and minimum right LE edema. Thromboembolic device (TED) stocking worn.

Table 1-1
Range of Motion

Left	Joint/Joint Complexes	Right	Comments
	Neck		
WFL	Flexion/extension	WFL	
WFL	Rotation	WFL	
WFL	Lateral flexion	WFL	
	Trunk		
Mod ↓	Flexion/extension	Mod	Secondary to postural deformities due to osteoporosis
Mod ↓	Rotation	Mod ↓	
Mod ↓	Lateral flexion	Mod ↓	
Mod ↓	Pelvic elevation	Mod ↓	
	Upper Extremities		
WNL	Scapular abd/add	WNL	
WNL	Scapular elevation	WNL	
WNL	Shoulder flexion/extension	WNL	
WNL	Shoulder abd/add	WNL	
WNL	Shoulder IR/ER	WNL	
WNL	Shoulder horizontal abd/add	WNL	
WNL	Elbow flexion/extension	WNL	
WNL	Forearm pronation/supination	WNL	
WNL	Wrist flexion/extension	WNL	
WNL	MCP flexion/extension	WNL	
WNL	PIP flexion/extension	WNL	
WNL	DIP flexion/extension	WNL	
WNL	Finger abd/add	WNL	
WNL	Thumb MCP flexion/extension	WNL	
WNL	Thumb ICP flexion/extension		
WNL	Thumb abd/add	WNL	
WNL	Thumb opposition	WNL	
	Lower Extremities		
30 degrees	SLR	50 degrees	
65/-20 degrees	Hip flexion/extension	110/5 degrees	

<u>Table 1-1 continued</u>

Left	Joint/Joint Complexes	Right	Comments
20/0 degrees	Hip abd/add	40/10 degrees	THP observed for LLE ROM testing. Limited by edema in sitting
0/18 degrees	Hip IR/ER	WNL/25 degrees	
90/-5 degrees	Knee flexion/extension	WNL	
WNL/0 degrees	Ankle plantar/dorsiflexion	WNL/0 degrees	
Min ↓	Foot eversion/inversion	Min ↓	
Min ↓	Great toe flexion/extension	Min ↓	
Min ↓	Toe MTP flexion/extension	Min ↓	
Min ↓	Toe IP flexion/extension	Min ↓	

Mod ↓ = moderate decrease; Min ↓ minimal decrease; abd = abduction; add = adduction; IR = internal rotation; ER = external rotation; MCP = metacarpophalangeal; PIP = proximal interphalangeal; DIP = distal interphalangeal; ICP = intermittent compression pump; WNL = within normal limits; WFL = within functional limits; SLR = straight leg raise; THP = total hip precautions; LLE = left lower extremity; ROM = range of motion.

8. *Balance*: Once attained, she can maintain sitting static balance and move through moderate active trunk excursions. She requires a walker to support standing at PWB status and requires moderate assistance to maintain static stance and ambulate 15 feet. Equilibrium and protective extension reactions appear slightly delayed but intact.

9. *Mobility*

Bed Mobility:

- *Rolling to the left: Not tested (NT) secondary to pain. Rolling to the right: Moderate assistance with abductor wedge*
- *Bridging: Moderate assistance*
- *Supine ↔ sit: Moderate assistance to maneuver left LE, move trunk, and maintain total hip precautions (THP)*
- *Equipment: Abductor wedge in place at all times in bed per doctor's order*

Transfers:

- *Sit ↔ stand using a standard walker (PWB on left LE): Moderate assistance for balance*
- *Bed ↔ wheelchair (w/c): Moderate assistance with moderate cues for technique*
- *W/c ↔ commode: Moderate assistance with moderate cues for technique*
- *Toilet: Maximum assistance with a three-in-one commode over the toilet*
- *Tub/shower: NT*
- *Car: NT*

10. *Gait*: Ambulation with walker 15 feet x 3 with shortness of breath (SOB) (respiratory rate [RR] increasing from 14 at rest to 22 with ambulation). Good PWB maintenance but poor LE clearance bilaterally in gait. Poor heel strike and increased hip flexion throughout gait cycle.

11. *Wheelchair mobility*: Minimum assistance primarily for cue for propulsion and maneuvering. She can propel her wheelchair 50 feet, then becomes SOB. Patient is independent with locking brakes prior to standing. She requires maximum assistance for leg rest placement and maneuvering.

12. *Self-care*

- *Feeding/equipment: Independent*
- *Bathing: Once seated in a wheelchair, the patient is able to bathe her upper body independently but requires moderate to maximum assistance for stand/wash.*
- *Grooming: She is independent in basic grooming tasks at a wheelchair level.*
- *Dressing: From a seated position she is able to dress her upper body but requires maximum assistance for LE dressing including stand-hike to don undergarments, pants, and for donning TED stockings and running shoes.*
- *Toileting: Requires maximum assistance to complete hygiene.*

13. *Home management*: This has not been assessed at this point, however it is clear that she will need assistance with home management tasks upon return home.

<u>Table 1-2</u>

Manual Muscle Test

Left	Muscle/Muscle Group	Right	Comments
	Neck		
WFL	Flexion/extension	WFL	
WFL	Rotation	WFL	
WFL	Lateral flexion	WFL	
	Trunk		
Mod↓	Flexion/extension	Mod↓	Not formally tested secondary to postural deformities, pain and THP observed functionally
Mod↓	Rotation	Mod↓	
Mod↓	Lateral flexion	Mod↓	
Mod↓	Pelvic elevation	Mod↓	
	Upper Extremities		
G	Scapular abd/add	G	
G	Scapular elevation	G	
G	Shoulder flexion/extension	G	
G	Shoulder abd/add	G	
G	Shoulder IR/ER	G	
G	Shoulder horizontal abd/add	G	
G+	Elbow flexion/extension	G+	
G+	Forearm pronation/supination	G+	
G+	Wrist flexion/extension	G+	
WNL	MCP flexion/extension	WNL	
WNL	PIP flexion/extension	WNL	
WNL	DIP flexion/extension	WNL	
WNL	Finger abd/add	WNL	
WNL	Thumb MCP flexion/extension	WNL	
WNL	Thumb ICP flexion/extension	WNL	
WNL	Thumb abd/add	WNL	
WNL	Thumb opposition	WNL	
	Lower Extremities		
P- /P-	Hip flexion/extension	F+/P+	Extension tested via modified bridge

<u>Table 1-2 continued</u>

Left	Muscle/Muscle Group	Right	Comments
P-/P	Hip abd/add	P+	
P/P	Hip IR/ER	F+/F+	
F-/F	Knee flexion/extension	F+/G-	Modified test in sitting
F+	Ankle plantar/dorsiflexion	G	
F+	Foot eversion/inversion	G	
G	Great toe flexion/extension	G	
G	Toe MTP flexion/extension	G	
G	Toe IP flexion/extension	G	

Mod ↓ = moderate decrease; abd = abduction; add = adduction; IR = internal rotation; ER = external rotation; MCP = metacarpophalangeal; PIP = proximal interphalangeal; DIP = distal interphalangeal; ICP = intermittent oppression pump; WNL = within normal limits; WFL = within functional limits; G = good (80%); G+ = good (90%); F = fair (50%); F+ = fair (60%); F- = fair (40%); P = poor (20%); P+ = poor (30%); P- = poor (10%).

PATIENT GOALS (PRIMARILY TO RETURN TO HER PRIOR LIVING SITUATION)

1. Independent bed mobility.
2. Independent self-care.
3. Independent transfers, including tub.
4. Independent ambulation with assistive device if necessary (preferably without).
5. Return to social activities.
6. Return to religious and family activities.

EXERCISES FOR THE OT AND PT STUDENT

Case #1: Josephine Walker

1. Using the Nagi scheme of disability, present the active pathology(ies), impairments, functional limitations, and disabilities for this case.
2. Do you think the patient's goals are realistic? Why or why not? If not, what strategies would you use to help the patient focus on more realistic goals?
3. Write an assessment and plan for the patient case(s) assigned. Include appropriate short-term and long-term goals.
4. Present a thorough plan of care for the case (ie, what specifically would you do with this patient and why?).
5. Design a treatment session lasting 30 minutes for this patient.

6. If both occupational and physical therapy were involved with this patient, what would you see as the role for each discipline to provide an appropriate, comprehensive treatment program? Consider the concepts of cotreatment and expert consultation in your answer.
7. Based upon the pathology that the patient exhibits and the individual impairments and functional limitations, do you think the patient will ever become totally "able" again? If not, which disabilities may remain?
8. What compensatory strategies might you teach the patient in this case?
9. What type(s) of durable medical equipment (DME) (orthotic, prosthetic, or adaptive equipment) might you prescribe and why?
10. What would you propose as an appropriate treatment frequency and length of stay for this patient in your treatment setting? Provide the rationale for your answer.
11. What modifications would you have to make to the plan of care if you received insurance approval for only one-half of the time requested and the patient did not want to fund therapy privately?
12. Which portion(s) of the plan of care would you delegate to an assistant? Which portion(s) to an aide/tech? Provide your rationale for your answer.
13. For physical therapy students: Using the *Guidelines for Practice*, what would be your physical therapy diagnosis for this patient?
14. What environment(s) would you choose for implementing your treatment activities?

15. What activities would you use to address this patient's values?

16. Who is this patient? What roles and activities are important to her?

17. What effects of the normal aging process might have an impact upon this patient's recovery process?

EXERCISES FOR THE ASSISTANT STUDENT

Case #1: Josephine Walker

1. Using the Nagi scheme of disability, present the active pathology(ies), impairments, functional limitations, and disabilities for this case.

2. Design a treatment session lasting 30 minutes for this patient.

3. If both occupational and physical therapy were involved with this patient, what would you see as the role for each discipline to provide an appropriate, comprehensive treatment program? Consider the concepts of cotreatment and expert consultation in your answer.

4. Based upon the pathology that the patient exhibits and the individual impairments and functional limitations, do you think the patient will ever become totally "able" again? If not, which disabilities may remain?

5. What compensatory strategies might you teach the patient in this case?

6. What type(s) of DME (orthotic, prosthetic, or adaptive equipment) might you prescribe and why?

7. Which portion(s) of the plan of care would you delegate to an aide/tech? Provide your rationale for your answer.

8. What environment(s) would you choose for implementing your treatment activities?

9. What activities would you use to address this patient's values?

10. Who is this patient? What roles and activities are important to her?

11. What effects of the normal aging process might have an impact upon this patient's recovery process?

Right Total Hip Replacement Secondary to Hip Fracture

Angela Lloyd is a 38-year-old single woman with Down syndrome. She lives in a fully accessible group home in the same suburban community as her biological family. Her daily routine consists of working Monday to Friday in a local publishing house. She has a job coach whom she shares with several other disabled workers. Her job involves packaging business manuals and other materials weighing no more than 7 pounds each. The company is located on the outskirts of town and has six stairs with bilateral railings to enter/exit. She thoroughly enjoys the financial and social aspects of her work.

Socially, Angela is an active participant in all group home activities and those with her family. She uses public transportation to visit her family and to go to the bowling alley. She has several active medical issues: osteoporosis, hypertension (HTN), and obesity. She was advised by her primary care physician to lose 35 to 40 pounds. She takes Lopressor (Novartis, East Hanover, NJ), Fosimax (for osteoporosis), and a multivitamin daily. She is quite independent in all areas of self-care. Angela easily becomes engrossed in social happenings and requires cues to initiate her daily routine. She states, "I don't want to miss anything."

While conversing and exiting the bus, Angela slipped and fell. This fall resulted in her receiving a subcapital fracture of her right hip. She underwent surgery for a total hip replacement (THR) and was referred to you in the home care setting for further rehabilitation after 11 days of acute inpatient rehabilitation. She has THP and an abduction wedge. Currently, she is having great difficulty recalling/incorporating her partial weightbearing status and precautions. Angela just wants everything to be back to the way it was.

The results of the initial evaluation are as follows:

1. *Perception*: WFL

Cognition:

- *Alert and Oriented x 2: She has difficulty defining the specifics of time.*

- *Attention: Her sustained attention is WFL. However, she has impaired divided attention.*

- *Concentration: Sustained concentration intact. Easily distracted when speaking and trying to perform a task.*

- *Memory: Long-term memory is functional. However, short-term memory and immediate recall are impaired, especially for abstract or multistep information.*

- *Sequencing: Able to sequence one to three new concrete steps, using verbal rehearsal. At times, she may require frequent cues.*

- *Ability to follow directions: Successfully follows demonstrated instructions. May require moderate cues if distracted.*

- *Initiation: WFL*

- *Insight/judgment: Impaired. Poor adherence to THP, including PWB.*

- *Problem solving: Impaired cause and effect (ie, following precautions and outcome).*

2. *Range of motion*: See Table 1-3.

3. *Sensation/pain*: Sensation appears WNL. Ms. Lloyd states she is in "a lot of pain" at rest and becomes quite agitated with passive range of motion (PROM) attempts nearing end ranges. She did appear to be quite pain-free during the mobility evaluation with the exception of gait using a standard walker. She expressed increased pain during weightbearing (WB) of right lower extremity (RLE).

Table 1-3

Range of Motion

Left	Joint/Joint Complexes	Right	Comments
	Neck		
¾ ROM	Flexion/extension	¾ ROM	
¾ ROM	Rotation	¾ ROM	
¾ ROM	Lateral flexion	¾ ROM	
	Trunk		
¾ ROM	Flexion/extension	¾ ROM	
¾ ROM	Rotation	¾ ROM	
¾ ROM	Lateral flexion	¾ ROM	
¾ ROM	Pelvic elevation	¾ ROM	
	Upper Extremities		
WNL	Scapular abd/add	WNL	
WNL	Scapular elevation	WNL	
WNL	Shoulder flexion/extension	WNL	
WNL	Shoulder abd/add	WNL	
WNL	Shoulder IR/ER	WNL	
WNL	Shoulder horizontal abd/add	WNL	
WNL	Elbow flexion/extension	WNL	
WNL	Forearm pronation/supination	WNL	
WNL	Wrist flexion/extension	WNL	
WNL	MCP flexion/extension	WNL	
WNL	PIP flexion/extension	WNL	
WNL	DIP flexion/extension	WNL	
WNL	Finger abd/add	WNL	
WNL	Thumb MCP flexion/extension	WNL	
WNL	Thumb ICP flexion/extension	WNL	
WNL	Thumb abd/add	WNL	
WNL	Thumb opposition	WNL	
	Lower Extremities		
WNL	SLR	70 to -10	
WNL	Hip flexion/extension	85 to -10	
WNL	Hip abd/add	25 to 0	
WNL	Hip IR/ER	0 to 30	

Table 1-3 continued

Left	Joint/Joint Complexes	Right	Comments
WNL	Knee flexion/extension	WNL	
WNL	Ankle plantar/dorsiflexion	WNL	
WNL	Foot eversion/inversion	WNL	
WNL	Great toe flexion/extension	WNL	
WNL	Toe MTP flexion/extension	WNL	
WNL	Toe IP flexion/extension	WNL	

abd = abduction; add = adduction; IR = internal rotation; ER = external rotation; MCP = metacarpophalangeal; PIP = proximal interphalangeal; DIP = distal interphalangeal; ICP = intermittent oppression pump; WNL = within normal limits; SLR = straight leg raise.

4. *Skin/edema*: Clean, closed suture with staples to be removed within 3 days.

5. *Balance*: Sitting balance is WNL for both static and dynamic positioning. Standing balance not assessed secondary to patient's inability to maintain safe weightbearing.

6. *Mobility*

Bed mobility:

- *Rolling: Minimum assistance with maximum cues, as patient is an active participant but does not incorporate*
- *Bridging: THP.*
- *Supine ↔ sit: THP.*
- *Equipment: Abductor wedge. Patient is noncompliant with wedge.*

Transfers:

- *Sit → stand: Minimum assistance with moderate to maximum cues secondary to difficulty maintaining weightbearing.*
- *Bed: Minimum assistance with moderate to maximum cues secondary to difficulty maintaining weightbearing.*
- *Chair: Minimum assistance with moderate to maximum cues secondary to difficulty maintaining weightbearing.*
- *Toilet: Minimum assistance with raised toilet and grab bars.*
- *Tub/shower: Minimum assistance with maximum cues to enter/exit stall shower.*
- *Car: NT.*

7. *Wheelchair mobility*: Supervised within the group home due to safety. She requires reminders to lock the chair's brakes.

8. *Gait/functional mobility*: Ms. Lloyd requires minimum assistance to ambulate 5 to 10 feet with her walker while trying to maintain PWB. She complains of increased RLE pain during ambulation.

9. *Self-care (right dominant):*

- *Feeding/equipment: Independent.*
- *Bathing: Independent upper body, seated. Maximum assistance for lower body secondary to inability to maintain THP.*
- *Grooming: Independent, seated.*
- *Dressing: Independent upper body, seated. Maximum assistance for lower body secondary to inability to maintain THP.*
- *Toileting: Maximum assistance secondary to inability to incorporate THP and weightbearing (WB) precautions during hygiene and clothing management.*
- *Home management: Assisting with tasks at wheelchair level. Volunteers to complete activities that may contraindicate THP.*
- *Leisure/community: Essentially homebound.*

PATIENT GOALS

1. Independent toileting.
2. Independent self-care.
3. Independent transfers without a device.
4. Independent ambulation without a device.
5. Return to her workshop position.
6. Return to her social activities with her family and in the group home.
7. Participate in household management tasks.

EXERCISES FOR THE OT AND PT STUDENT

Case #2: Angela Lloyd

1. Using the Nagi scheme of disability, present the active pathology(ies), impairments, functional limitations, and disabilities for this case.

2. Do you think the patient's goals are realistic? Why or why not? If not, what strategies would you use to help the patient focus on more realistic goals?

3. Write an assessment and plan for the patient case(s) assigned. Include appropriate short-term and long-term goals.

4. Present a thorough plan of care for the case (ie, what specifically would you do with this patient and why?)

5. Design a treatment session lasting 30 minutes for this patient.

6. If both occupational and physical therapy were involved with this patient, what would you see as the role for each discipline to provide an appropriate, comprehensive treatment program? Consider the concepts of cotreatment and expert consultation in your answer.

7. Based upon the pathology that the patient exhibits and the individual impairments and functional limitations, do you think the patient will ever become totally "able" again? If not, which disabilities may remain?

8. What compensatory strategies might you teach the patient in this case?

9. What type(s) of DME (orthotic, prosthetic, or adaptive equipment) might you prescribe and why?

10. What would you propose as an appropriate treatment frequency and length of stay for this patient in your treatment setting? Provide the rationale for your answer.

11. What modifications would you have to make to the plan of care if you received insurance approval for only one-half of the time requested and the patient did not want to fund therapy privately?

12. Which portion(s) of the plan of care would you delegate to an assistant? Which portion(s) to an aide/tech? Provide your rationale for your answer.

13. For physical therapy students: Using the *Guidelines for Practice*, what would be your physical therapy diagnosis for this patient?

14. What environment(s) would you choose for implementing your treatment activities?

15. What activities would you use to address this patient's values?

16. Who is this patient? What roles and activities are important to her?

17. Design a cueing system to address this patient's poor carryover.

EXERCISES FOR ASSISTANT STUDENT

Case #2: Angela Lloyd

1. Using the Nagi scheme of disability, present the active pathology(ies), impairments, functional limitations, and disabilities for this case.

2. Design a treatment session lasting 30 minutes for this patient.

3. If both occupational and physical therapy were involved with this patient, what would you see as the role for each discipline to provide an appropriate, comprehensive treatment program? Consider the concepts of cotreatment and expert consultation in your answer.

4. Based upon the pathology that the patient exhibits and the individual impairments and functional limitations, do you think the patient will ever become totally "able" again? If not, which disabilities may remain?

5. What compensatory strategies might you teach the patient in this case?

6. What type(s) of DME (orthotic, prosthetic, or adaptive equipment) might you prescribe and why?

7. Which portion(s) of the plan of care would you delegate to an aide/tech? Provide your rationale for your answer.

8. What environment(s) would you choose for implementing your treatment activities?

9. What activities would you use to address this patient's values?

10. Who is this patient? What roles and activities are important to her?

11. Design a cueing system to address this patient's poor carryover.

Multiple Fractures

David Jones is a 29-year-old newlywed who fell off of his roof while making a repair. He is a carpenter by trade and his wife is a full-time travel agent. They live on the second floor of a two-family house that David owns with his sister. His sister and her family occupy the first floor unit. There are 24 stairs to enter David's apartment, but once inside there are no other obstacles. The bathroom is tiled and has sliding shower doors. The kitchen is galley style with all meals eaten in the dining room.

Mr. Jones led an active life. He played rugby and golfed weekly. He has no significant medical history; however, from his fall, he sustained a right comminuted tibial fracture with external fixation and a right distal radius fracture with a cast applied. He is nonweightbearing (NWB) on both the right wrist and lower extremity for 6 to 8 weeks. He is receiving Darvocet (Eli Lilly, Indianapolis, Ind) prn.

He is referred for evaluation and treatment in acute care with the plan being for him to be discharged home within several days. Your department will treat him in acute care and will then continue his services through your home health department.

The results of the initial evaluation are as follows:

1. *Cognition/perception*: WNL

2. *ROM*: See Tables 1-4 and Table 1-5.

3. *Strength*: See Table 1-6.

4. *Sensation/pain*: Intact sensation with hypersensitivity to light touch on right palmar surface and able to sense light touch input only five out of 10 trials on right plantar surface of foot. Patient reports throbbing pain through both fracture sites. At rest, patient has right wrist pain of 2, during AROM, of 3 on a 1 to 10 scale. His RLE is a 4 at rest and a 7 with AROM and MMT. This is limiting his ability to perform during strength testing to his true abilities.

5. *Skin/edema*: Positional edema present. Pin sites are clean and infection free.

6. *Balance*: Static sit is WNL, and dynamic sit is WFL during moderate excursions. Pain is a limiting factor. Static stand is F+ with safety as an issue during transfers and ambulation.

7. *Mobility*

Bed mobility:

- *Rolling: Rolls to the right with minimum assistance. Rolls to the left with maximum assistance.*
- *Bridging: Minimum assistance with rails and LLE.*
- *Supine ↔ sit: Minimum assistance with slow, deliberate movement of RLE.*
- *Equipment: Half rails.*

Transfers:

- *Sit → stand: Moderate assistance with right platform crutch and left axillary crutch for positioning, balance, and maintenance of NWB of RLE.*
- *Bed ↔ stand: Moderate assistance with right platform crutch and left axillary crutch for positioning, balance, and maintenance of NWB of RLE.*
- *Chair ↔ stand (with armrests): Moderate assistance with right platform crutch and left axillary crutch for positioning, balance, and maintenance of NWB of RLE.*
- *Toilet ↔ stand (with versa frame): Moderate assistance with right platform crutch and left axillary crutch for positioning, balance, and maintenance of NWB of RLE.*
- *Tub/shower ↔ stand (uses seat): Moderate assistance with right platform crutch and left axillary crutch for positioning, balance, and maintenance of NWB of RLE.*
- *Car: To be evaluated.*

8. *Wheelchair mobility*: Patient is easily able to learn how to use a one arm drive wheelchair with elevating swing away leg rest for RLE. He requires minimum cues to propel and maneuver but moderate assistance to maneuver the right leg rest. He can propel the chair > 200 feet straight without fatigue.

9. *Gait/functional mobility*: Patient is able to ambulate 15 feet x 3 with minimum to moderate assistance for balance and cues to maintain NWB of RLE. Gait is very slow and painful, primarily in his RLE. He uses a right platform crutch and a left axillary crutch. Stairs not tested.

10. *Self-care (right dominant):*

- *Feeding/equipment: Requires set-up for all bilateral activities. Is managing, but slowly.*
- *Bathing: Bedside, chair level with minimum assistance for upper body with the exception of dependence for left upper extremity (LUE). Lower body requires moderate assistance and maximum assistance for RLE. Using lateral weight shifting for peri-area. States he wants to have privacy during all bathing activities. Extremities experience increased pain after bathing.*
- *Grooming: Set-up necessary for all bilateral activities. Is able to use an electric razor but prefers a straight edge.*
- *Dressing: Chair level—Overhead shirt with minimum assistance. Pants and footwear require maximum assistance.*
- *Toileting: See transfers. Able to complete hygiene.*
- *Home management: To be evaluated.*
- *Leisure/community: Plans to return to prior activities.*

PATIENT GOALS

1. Independent self-care.
2. Independent transfers without a device.
3. Independent ambulation without a device.
4. Return to work.
5. Return to recreational rugby.

EXERCISES FOR THE OT AND PT STUDENT

Case #3: David Jones

1. Using the Nagi scheme of disability, present the active pathology(ies), impairments, functional limitations, and disabilities for this case.

2. Do you think the patient's goals are realistic? Why or why not? If not, what strategies would you use to help the patient focus on more realistic goals?

3. Write an assessment and plan for the patient case(s) assigned. Include appropriate short-term and long-term goals.

4. Present a thorough plan of care for the case (ie, what specifically would you do with this patient and why?)

5. Design a treatment session lasting 30 minutes for this patient.

<u>Table 1-4</u>

Range of Motion

Left	Joint/Joint Complexes	Right	Comments
	Neck		
WNL	Flexion/extension	WNL	
WNL	Rotation	WNL	
WNL	Lateral flexion	WNL	
	Trunk		
WNL	Flexion/extension	WNL	
WNL	Rotation	WNL	
WNL	Lateral flexion	WNL	
WNL	Pelvic elevation	WNL	
	Upper Extremities		
WNL	Scapular abd/add	WNL	
WNL	Scapular elevation	WNL	
WNL	Shoulder flexion/extension	WNL	
WNL	Shoulder abd/add	WNL	
WNL	Shoulder IR/ER	WNL	
WNL	Shoulder horizontal abd/add	WNL	
WNL	Elbow flexion/extension	≈ 1/2	
WNL	Forearm pronation/supination	NT	
WNL	Wrist flexion/extension	NT	
WNL	MCP flexion/extension	NT	
WNL	PIP flexion/extension	NT	
WNL	DIP flexion/extension	NT	
WNL	Finger abd/add	NT	
WNL	Thumb MCP flexion/extension	NT	
WNL	Thumb ICP flexion/extension	NT	
WNL	Thumb abd/add	NT	
WNL	Thumb opposition	NT	
	Lower Extremities		
WNL	SLR	WNL	
WNL	Hip flexion/extension	WNL	
WNL	Hip abd/add	WNL	
WNL	Hip IR/ER	WNL	

Table 1-4 continued

Left	Joint/Joint Complexes	Right	Comments
WNL	Knee flexion/extension	60/-10	
WNL	Ankle plantar/dorsiflexion	10/-10	
WNL	Foot eversion/inversion	WNL	
WNL	Great Toe flexion/extension	WNL	
WNL	Toe MTP flexion/extension	WNL	
WNL	Toe IP flexion/extension	WNL	

abd = abduction; add = adduction; IR = internal rotation; ER = external rotation; MCP = metacarpophalangeal; PIP = proximal interphalangeal; DIP = distal interphalangeal; ICP = intermittent compression pump; WNL = within normal limits; SLR = straight leg raise.

Table 1-5

Active Range of Motion

Left	Joint/Joint Complexes	Right	Comments
	Neck		
WNL	Flexion/extension	WNL	
WNL	Rotation	WNL	
WNL	Lateral flexion	WNL	
	Trunk		
WNL	Flexion/extension	WNL	
WNL	Rotation	WNL	
WNL	Lateral flexion	WNL	
WNL	Pelvic elevation	WNL	
	Upper Extremities		
WNL	Scapular abd/add	WNL	
WNL	Scapular elevation	WNL	
WNL	Shoulder flexion/extension	WNL	
WNL	Shoulder abd/add	WNL	
WNL	Shoulder IR/ER	WNL	
WNL	Shoulder horizontal abd/add	WNL	
WNL	Elbow flexion/extension	≈ 1/4	
WNL	Forearm pronation/supination	NT	

Table 1-5 continued

Left	Joint/Joint Complexes	Right	Comments
WNL	Wrist flexion/extension	NT	
WNL	MCP flexion/extension	NT	
WNL	PIP flexion/extension	Initiates	
WNL	DIP flexion/extension	≈ 1/2	
WNL	Finger abd/add	Not Tested	
WNL	Thumb MCP flexion/extension	Initiates	
WNL	Thumb ICP flexion/extension	Initiates	
WNL	Thumb abd/add	≈ 1/4	Painful
WNL	Thumb opposition	≈ 1/4	
	Lower Extremities		
WNL	SLR	WNL	
WNL	Hip flexion/extension	WNL	
WNL	Hip abd/add	WNL	
WNL	Hip IR/ER	WNL	
WNL	Knee flexion/extension	≈ 1/4	Painful
WNL	Ankle plantar/dorsiflexion	30/0	Painful
WNL	Foot eversion/inversion	5/10	Painful
WNL	Great toe flexion/extension	Initiates ROM	Painful
WNL	Toe MTP flexion/extension	Initiates ROM	Painful
WNL	Toe IP flexion/extension	Initiates ROM	Painful

abd = abduction; add = adduction; IR = internal rotation; ER = external rotation; MCP = metacarpophalangeal; PIP = proximal interphalangeal; DIP = distal interphalangeal; ICP = intermittent compression pump; WNL = within normal limits; SLR = straight leg raise.

Table 1-6

Manual Muscle Test

Left	Muscle/Muscle Group	Right	Comments
	Neck		
N	Flexion/extension	N	
N	Rotation	N	
N	Lateral flexion	N	

Table 1-6 continued

Left	Muscle/Muscle Group	Right	Comments
	Trunk		
N	Flexion/extension	N	
N	Rotation	N	
N	Lateral flexion	N	
N	Pelvic elevation	N	
	Upper Extremities		
N	Scapular abd/add	N	
N	Scapular elevation	N	
N	Shoulder flexion/extension	F+	Patient reports pain with any resistance
N	Shoulder abd/add	P	
N	Shoulder IR/ER	F/P	
N	Shoulder horizontal abd/add	P	
N	Elbow flexion/extension	F-	
N	Forearm pronation/supination	NT	
N	Wrist flexion/extension	NT	
N	MCP flexion/extension	NT	
N	PIP flexion/extension	NT	
N	DIP flexion/extension	NT	
N	Finger abd/add	NT	
N	Thumb MCP flexion/extension	NT	
N	Thumb ICP flexion/extension	NT	
N	Thumb abd/add	NT	
N	Thumb opposition	NT	
	Lower Extremities		
N	Hip flexion/extension	G/G-	Radiating pain
N	Hip abd/add	F-/F	Radiating pain
N	Hip IR/ER	F-	Radiating pain
N	Knee flexion/extension	P	Radiating pain
N	Ankle plantar/dorsiflexion	P	Radiating pain
N	Foot eversion/inversion	P	Radiating pain

Table 1-6 continued

Left	Muscle/Muscle Group	Right	Comments
N	Great toe flexion/extension	F-	Radiating pain
N	Toe MTP flexion/extension	F-	Radiating pain
N	Toe IP flexion/extension	F	Radiating pain

abd = abduction; add = adduction; IR = internal rotation; ER = external rotation; MCP = metacarpophalangeal; PIP = proximal interphalangeal; DIP = distal interphalangeal; ICP = intermittent oppression pump; WNL = within normal limits; SLR = straight leg raise.

6. If both occupational and physical therapy were involved with this patient, what would you see as the role for each discipline to provide an appropriate, comprehensive treatment program? Consider the concepts of cotreatment and expert consultation in your answer.

7. Based upon the pathology that the patient exhibits and the individual impairments and functional limitations, do you think the patient will ever become totally "able" again? If not, which disabilities may remain?

8. What compensatory strategies might you teach the patient in this case?

9. What type(s) of DME (orthotic, prosthetic, or adaptive equipment) might you prescribe and why?

10. What would you propose as an appropriate treatment frequency and length of stay for this patient in your treatment setting? Provide the rationale for your answer.

11. What modifications would you have to make to the plan of care if you received insurance approval for only one-half of the time requested and the patient did not want to fund therapy privately?

12. Which portion(s) of the plan of care would you delegate to an assistant? Which portion(s) to an aide/tech? Provide your rationale for your answer.

13. For physical therapy students: Using the *Guidelines for Practice*, what would be your physical therapy diagnosis for this patient?

14. What environment(s) would you choose for implementing your treatment activities?

15. What activities would you use to address this patient's values?

16. Who is this patient? What roles and activities are important to him?

17. Considering his recent marriage and new stressors, how would you want to engage his spouse in the treatment process? (Consider the fact that for financial reasons she can only take a 2-week leave of absence from work).

18. How do you address patient privacy issues, especially when the patient is adamant about maintaining his privacy at all times?

EXERCISES FOR THE ASSISTANT STUDENT

Case #2: David Jones

1. Using the Nagi scheme of disability, present the active pathology(ies), impairments, functional limitations, and disabilities for this case.

2. Design a treatment session lasting 30 minutes for this patient.

3. If both occupational and physical therapy were involved with this patient, what would you see as the role for each discipline to provide an appropriate, comprehensive treatment program? Consider the concepts of cotreatment and expert consultation in your answer.

4. Based upon the pathology that the patient exhibits and the individual impairments and functional limitations, do you think the patient will ever become totally "able" again? If not, which disabilities may remain?

5. What compensatory strategies might you teach the patient in this case?

6. What type(s) of DME (orthotic, prosthetic, or adaptive equipment) might you prescribe and why?

7. Which portion(s) of the plan of care would you delegate to an aide/tech? Provide your rationale for your answer.

8. What environment(s) would you choose for implementing your treatment activities?

9. What activities would you use to address this patient's values?

10. Who is this patient? What roles and activities are important to him?

11. Considering his recent marriage and new stressors, how would you want to engage his spouse in the treatment process? (Consider the fact that for financial reasons she can only take a 2-week leave of absence from work).

12. How do you address patient privacy issues, especially when the patient is adamant about maintaining his privacy at all times?

NEUROLOGY

Guillain-Barré Syndrome

Joseph Taylor is a 48-year-old electrician who lives with his wife and 14-year-old daughter in a single family home that they have owned for 10 years. He is a typical husband and father, independent in all activities of daily living and devoted to his family. He particularly enjoys his daily 5-mile run with his daughter, who is training to make the high school cross country team next year. He also likes spending some time on his own fishing at the local lake. He and his wife enjoy a weekly night out every Friday. He is the primary caretaker of the house and yard, often doing the major repairs such as painting and renovations.

He battled a bout of flu during the winter and, just as he was feeling better, he began to experience significant generalized muscle weakness, malaise, fever, and some parasthesia in his hands. Initially, he thought he was having a recurrence of the flu.

His symptoms rapidly progressed over a 48-hour period to the point that he was having difficulty breathing. He contacted his physician who told him to go to the emergency room and that he would meet him there. After examination and some laboratory tests, his physician diagnosed him with Guillain-Barré syndrome and he was admitted to the intensive care unit (ICU). The progressive nature of the acute phase of this disorder resulted in his respiratory status becoming so compromised that he was intubated after 12 hours in the ICU. He began to regain some strength and was extubated 2 days after his admission. He spent 4 more days on the neurological floor of the hospital and was then discharged to your inpatient rehabilitation facility with orders for OT and PT evaluation and treatment to regain maximum mobility.

He presents to you in the clinic with the following findings:

1. *Significant past medical history*: Without significant past medical history (PMH). He is status post (s/p) appendectomy 25 years ago, and s/p hernia repair 5 years ago.

2. *Medications:* Tylenol prn for occasional headaches and overall body aches due to immobility.

3. *Cognition/perception*: He is alert and oriented x 3 without cognitive or perceptual issues.

4. *Sensation/tone*: He reports parasthesia of the feet and hands. He is able to correctly identify six of 10 sensory stimuli for light touch and pain/temperature in all distal extremities. Proprioception is intact. Trunk and extremity musculature are moderately hypotonic, with the greatest hypotonicity at distal muscles.

5. *ROM*: See Table 2-1.

6. *Strength*: See Table 2-2.

7. *Balance*: He is able to sit on the edge of the bed with moderate assistance and can hold his head up independently for 3 to 5 minutes, then his neck and trunk muscles fatigue.

8. *Pain*: At rest he reports resting pain and stiffness due to immobility as a 3 on a 1 to 10 scale. The stiffness is especially pronounced in the low back muscles.

9. *Skin/edema*: Intact skin integrity. Moderate distal LE edema. TED stocking worn.

10. *Mobility*

Bed mobility:

- *Rolling: Moderate assistance.*
- *Bridging: Maximum assistance.*
- *Supine ↔ sit: Moderate assistance.*
- *Equipment: Uses bed handle to facilitate sit to supine.*

10. *Transfers*: Transfers require maximum assistance for bed to wheelchair using a slide board.

<u>Table 2-1</u>
Transfers

Left	Joint/Joint Complexes	Right	Comments
	Neck		
WNL	Flexion/extension	WNL	
WNL	Rotation	WNL	
WNL	Lateral flexion	WNL	
	Trunk		
WNL	Flexion/extension	WNL	
WNL	Rotation	WNL	
WNL	Lateral flexion	WNL	
WNL	Pelvic elevation	WNL	
	Upper Extremities		
WNL	Scapular abd/add	WNL	
WNL	Scapular elevation	WNL	
WNL	Shoulder flexion/extension	WNL	
WNL	Shoulder abd/add	WNL	
WNL	Shoulder IR/ER	WNL	
WNL	Shoulder horizontal abd/add	WNL	
WNL	Elbow flexion/extension	WNL	
WNL	Forearm pronation/supination	WNL	
WNL	Wrist flexion/extension	WNL	
WNL	MCP flexion/extension	WNL	
WNL	PIP flexion/extension	WNL	
WNL	DIP flexion/extension	WNL	
WNL	Finger abd/add	WNL	
WNL	Thumb MCP flexion/extension	WNL	
WNL	Thumb ICP flexion/extension	WNL	
WNL	Thumb abd/add	WNL	
WNL	Thumb opposition	WNL	
	Lower Extremities		
70 degrees	SLR	70 degrees	
WNL	Hip flexion/extension	WNL	
30 degrees/WNL	Hip abd/add	34 degrees/WNL	
WNL	Hip IR/ER	WNL	

Table 2-1 continued

Left	Joint/Joint Complexes	Right	Comments
WNL	Knee flexion/extension	WNL	
WNL/-5 degrees	Ankle plantar/dorsiflexion	WNL/0 degrees	
WNL	Foot eversion/inversion	WNL	
WNL	Great toe flexion/extension	WNL	
WNL	Toe MTP flexion/extension	WNL	
WNL	Toe IP flexion/extension	WNL	

abd = abduction; add = adduction; IR = internal rotation; ER = external rotation; MCP = metacarpophalangeal; PIP = proximal interphalangeal; DIP = distal interphalangeal; ICP = intermittent compression pump; WNL = within normal limits; SLR = straight leg raise.

Table 2-2

Manual Muscle Test

Left	Muscle/Muscle Group	Right	Comments
	Neck		
F/F+	Flexion/extension	F/F+	Tested functionally in sitting, muscle fatigue is a significant issue for function
F/F+	Rotation	F/F+	
F/F+	Lateral flexion	F/F+	
	Trunk		
P/P+	Flexion/extension	P/P+	
P/P+	Rotation	P/P+	
P/P+	Lateral flexion	P/P+	
NT	Pelvic elevation	NT	
	Upper Extremities		
F/F+	Scapular abd/add	F/F+	
F/F+	Scapular elevation	F/F+	
F/F+	Shoulder flexion/extension	F/F+	
F/F+	Shoulder abd/add	F/F+	
F/F+	Shoulder IR/ER	F/F+	
F+/F+	Shoulder horizontal abd/add	F+/F+	
F/F+	Elbow flexion/extension	F/F+	
F/F+	Forearm pronation/supination	F/F+	

Table 2-2 continued

Left	Muscle/Muscle Group	Right	Comments
P+/F-	Wrist flexion/extension	P+/F-	
P+/F-	MCP flexion/extension	P+/F-	Poor grasp for functional activities
P+/F-	PIP flexion/extension	P+/F-	
P+/F-	DIP flexion/extension	P+/F-	
P+/F-	Finger abd/add	P+/F-	
P+/F-	Thumb MCP flexion/extension	P+/F-	
P+/F-	Thumb ICP flexion/extension	P+/F-	
P+/F-	Thumb abd/add	P+/F-	
P+/F-	Thumb opposition	P+/F-	
	Lower Extremities		
P+	Hip flexion/extension	P+	
P+	Hip abd/add	P+	
P+	Hip IR/ER	P+	
P+	Knee flexion/extension	P+	
P	Ankle plantar/dorsiflexion	P	
P	Foot eversion/inversion	P	
P	Great toe flexion/extension	P	
P	Toe MTP flexion/extension	P	
P	Toe IP flexion/extension	P	

abd = abduction; add = adduction; IR = internal rotation; ER = external rotation; MCP = metacarpophalangeal; PIP = proximal interphalangeal; DIP = distal interphalangeal; ICP = intermittent oppression pump; WNL = within normal limits; WFL = within functional limits; G = good (80%); G+ = good (90%); F = fair (50%); F+ = fair (60%); F- = fair (40%); P = poor (20%); P+ = poor (30%); P- = poor (10%).

Transfers:

- *Sit → stand: Unable at present.*
- *Bed ↔ w/c: Maximum assistance with slide board.*
- *w/c ↔ commode: Maximum assistance with slide board. Uses drop arm commode.*
- *Toilet ↔ w/c: NT*
- *Tub/shower ↔ w/c: NT*
- *Car ↔ w/c: Maximum assistance x 2.*

11. *Wheelchair mobility*: This patient is able to propel his wheelchair 25 to 50 feet independently on open level surfaces with adapted wheels to decrease reliance on grasp for propulsion. He then fatigues and requires total assistance for wheelchair mobility.

12. *Gait*: This patient is unable to ambulate at this time.

13. *Functional mobility*: He is dependent for all functional mobility tasks at a manual wheelchair level. He is unable to drive.

14. *Self-care*: He is dependent for all aspects of self-care, including bathing, grooming, dressing, feeding, and toileting.

15. *Home management*: This patient is dependent for all home management tasks at present.

PATIENT GOALS (PRIMARILY TO RETURN TO HIS PRIOR LIVING SITUATION)

1. Independent bed mobility.
2. Independent transfers.
3. Independent toileting.
4. Independent self-care.
5. Independent ambulation with assistive device if necessary, then follow-up therapy to return to ambulation without a device.
6. Return to social activities without the need for assistance.
7. Return to driving.
8. Return to previous leisure activities.
9. Return to all home management tasks.

EXERCISES FOR THE OT AND PT STUDENT

Case # 4: Joseph Taylor

1. Using the Nagi scheme of disability, present the active pathology(ies), impairments, functional limitations, and disabilities for this case.
2. Do you think the patient's goals are realistic? Why or why not? If not, what strategies would you use to help the patient focus on more realistic goals?
3. Write an assessment and plan for the patient case(s) assigned. Include appropriate short-term and long-term goals.
4. Present a thorough plan of care for the case (ie, what specifically would you do with this patient and why?).
5. Design a treatment session lasting 30 minutes for this patient.
6. If both occupational and physical therapy were involved with this patient, what would you see as the role for each discipline to provide an appropriate, comprehensive treatment program? Consider the concepts of cotreatment and expert consultation in your answer.
7. Based upon the pathology that the patient exhibits and the individual impairments and functional limitations, do you think the patient will ever become totally "able" again? If not, which disabilities may remain?
8. What compensatory strategies might you teach the patient in this case?
9. What type(s) of DME (orthotic, prosthetic, or adaptive equipment) might you prescribe and why?
10. What would you propose as an appropriate treatment frequency and length of stay for this patient in your treatment setting? Provide the rationale for your answer.
11. What modifications would you have to make to the plan of care if you received insurance approval for only one-half of the time requested and the patient did not want to fund therapy privately?
12. Which portion(s) of the plan of care would you delegate to an assistant? Which portion(s) to an aide/tech? Provide your rationale for your answer.
13. For physical therapy students: Using the *Guidelines for Practice*, what would be your physical therapy diagnosis for this patient?
14. What environment(s) would you choose for implementing your treatment activities?
15. What activities would you use to address this patient's values?
16. Who is this patient? What roles and activities are important to him?

EXERCISES FOR THE ASSISTANT STUDENT

Case #4: Joseph Taylor

1. Using the Nagi scheme of disability, present the active pathology(ies), impairments, functional limitations, and disabilities for this case.
2. Design a treatment session lasting 30 minutes for this patient.
3. If both occupational and physical therapy were involved with this patient, what would you see as the role for each discipline to provide an appropriate, comprehensive treatment program? Consider the concepts of cotreatment and expert consultation in your answer.
4. Based upon the pathology that the patient exhibits, and the individual impairments and functional limitations, do you think the patient will ever become totally "able" again? If not, which disabilities may remain?
5. What compensatory strategies might you teach the patient in this case?
6. What type(s) of DME (orthotic, prosthetic, or adaptive equipment) might you prescribe and why?
7. Which portion(s) of the plan of care would you delegate to an aide/tech? Provide your rationale for your answer.
8. What environment(s) would you choose for implementing your treatment activities?
9. What activities would you use to address this patient's values?
10. Who is this patient? What roles and activities are important to him?

Parkinson's Disease

Frances Littleton is a 78-year-old woman who lives with her husband of 60 years in a small, cape-style home in New England.

For the past 20 years, her focus in life has been her battle with Parkinson's disease. For Frances, this has been slowly progressive over the years, resulting in her having to change roles from the primary homemaker and child care provider for her two grandchildren, now ages 16 and 18, to, as she puts it, "...someone who just sits around the house and waits for others to do for me." She has had to also battle significant depression, which has resulted from her decline in function and current disability. She often states that "Sometimes I just don't care anymore. It would be easier if I was no longer around." Frances is followed by a social worker who provides home visits for her twice a month. She also attends the monthly meeting of the Parkinson's support group in her area.

Last month, Frances noted an exacerbation of her signs and symptoms, which ultimately resulted in her falling four times in that time period. Two falls occurred when Frances attempted to stand from her favorite armchair one when getting out of bed, and one when she was carrying a watering can to water her plants. Although Frances was not overly concerned about this, her husband became quite alarmed, knowing that he could not continue to care for her at home if she were to continue to fall and perhaps seriously injure herself. Her husband contacted her neurologist about the decline in her function and, after a visit to him last week, was pleased that he changed her medications and referred her for physical and occupational therapy in the home care setting.

She presents to you in the clinic with the following findings:

1. *Significant past medical history*: Pallidotomy 15 years earlier, pacemaker placement 4 years ago, CHF, and depression.

2. *Medications*: The patient's antiparkinsonian medications consisted of selegiline HCL (Eldepryl) and carbidopa/levodopa (Sinemet). She also takes Lasix (Hoescht, Kansas City, Mo) and Elavil (Merck, West Point, Pa).

3. *Cognition/perception*: WFL except for mild dressing apraxia and depth perception deficits noted, especially during ambulation on uneven surfaces or stairs.

Cognition:

- *Alert and oriented x 3*
- *Attention: WNL for short timespans (5 minutes). Patient has difficulty attending to an entire home care session without loss of attention.*
- *Concentration: Minimally impaired sustained concentration.*
- *Memory: Intact long-term memory but limitation in short-term and recent memory for function in her environment. She relies heavily on her husband for support in this area.*
- *Sequencing: Able to complete two-and three-step tasks but breaks down with complex tasks.*
- *Ability to follow directions: Limited due to memory and concentration deficits.*

- *Initiation: Poor task initiation. Her husband reports that he must cue her to initiate many basic functional tasks such as dressing, light meal prep, and feeding (ie, preparing and eating a cold breakfast in the am).*
- *Insight/judgment: Moderately limited with patient often taking chances with her safety, such as attempting transfers without assistance or outdoor ambulation without waiting for her husband's support. She does not fully understand her physical deficits. This is further complicated by her depression.*
- *Problem solving: Fair ability to solve basic functional problems, however patient may be at risk if left alone to solve a complex problem (eg, patient was unable to state what she would do if her husband became too ill to get out of bed in the morning).*

4. *Strength*: See Table 2-3.

5. *ROM*: See Table 2-4.

6. *Neurological*: Sensation is intact for light touch, pain, temperature, deep pressure, proprioception, and kinesthesia. Resting tremor is slight and does not impair function. She has moderate truncal rigidity. Balance in sitting was within normal limits for static stability. In standing she is able to tolerate moderate perturbations to static standing when she expected the challenge, but lost her balance four of 10 trials when perturbations were unexpected. She demonstrates a decrease in balance during movement transitions such as ambulation, sit to stand, and when sitting on the edge of the bed to dress her lower extremities. She does not demonstrate any signs of autonomic nervous system dysfunction, which would cause instability at present (ie, orthostatic hypotension or drop attacks).

7. *Pain*: Without complaints of pain in any area.

8. *Skin/edema*: Skin is intact but appears thin and fragile. This patient wears TED stockings for edema control secondary to a history of mild edema resulting from her chronic CHF. Edema at this time is minimal in the feet and ankles only.

9. *Mobility*

Bed mobility:

- *Rolling: Minimum assistance secondary to truncal rigidity with cues for technique.*
- *Bridging: Minimum assistance secondary to truncal rigidity with cues for technique.*
- *Supine ↔ sit: Minimum assistance secondary to truncal rigidity with cues for technique.*
- *Equipment: None used at present.*

Transfers:

- *Sit → stand: Supervised from firm surface with arms. Minimum assistance from low, soft armchair (her favorite).*
- *Bed ↔ chair: Minimum assistance with cues for technique.*

<u>Table 2-3</u>

Manual Muscle Test

Left	Muscle/Muscle Group	Right	Comments
	Neck		
WFL	Flexion/extension	WFL	
WFL	Rotation	WFL	
WFL	Lateral flexion	WFL	
	Trunk		
Mod ↓	Flexion/extension	Mod ↓	
Mod ↓	Rotation	Mod ↓	
Mod ↓	Lateral flexion	Mod ↓	
Mod ↓	Pelvic elevation	Mod ↓	
	Upper Extremities		
WFL	Scapular abd/add	WFL	
WFL	Scapular elevation	WFL	
WFL	Shoulder flexion/extension	WFL	
WFL	Shoulder abd/add	WFL	
WFL	Shoulder IR/ER	WFL	
WFL	Shoulder horizontal abd/add	WFL	
WFL	Elbow flexion/extension	WFL	
WFL	Forearm pronation/supination	WFL	
WFL	Wrist flexion/extension	WFL	
WFL	MCP flexion/extension	WFL	
WFL	PIP flexion/extension	WFL	
WFL	DIP flexion/extension	WFL	
WFL	Finger abd/add	WFL	
WFL	Thumb MCP flexion/extension	WFL	
WFL	Thumb ICP flexion/extension	WFL	
WFL	Thumb abd/add	WFL	
WFL	Thumb opposition	WFL	
	Lower Extremities		
F+/F-	Hip flexion/extension	F+/F-	
P+/P+	Hip abd/add	P+/P+	
F+/F+	Hip IR/ER	F+/F+	
F+/G-	Knee flexion/extension	F+/G-	

Table 2-3 continued

Left	Muscle/Muscle Group	Right	Comments
F+/G-	Ankle plantar/dorsiflexion	F+/G-	Dorsiflexion with limited ROM
WFL	Foot eversion/inversion	WFL	
WFL	Great toe flexion/extension	WFL	
WFL	Toe MTP flexion/extension	WFL	
WFL	Toe IP flexion/extension	WFL	

Mod↓ = moderate decrease; abd = abduction; add = adduction; IR = internal rotation; ER = external rotation; MCP = metacarpophalangeal; PIP = proximal interphalangeal; DIP = distal interphalangeal; ICP = intermittent oppression pump; WNL = within normal limits; WFL = within functional limits; SLR = straight leg raise; G = good (80%); G+ = good (90%); F = fair (50%); F+ = fair (60%); F- = fair (40%); P = poor (20%); P+ = poor (30%); P- = poor (10%).

Table 2-4

Range of Motion

Left	Joint/Joint Complexes	Right	Comments
	Neck		
Mod ↓	Flexion/extension	Mod ↓	
Mod ↓	Rotation	Mod ↓	
Mod ↓	Lateral flexion	Mod ↓	
	Trunk		
WFL/mod ↓	Flexion/extension	WFL/mod ↓	
Min ↓	Rotation	Min ↓	
Mod ↓	Lateral flexion	Mod ↓	
Mod ↓	Pelvic elevation	Mod ↓	
	Upper Extremities		
WFL	Scapular abd/add	WFL	
WFL	Scapular elevation	WFL	
150 degrees/WNL	Shoulder flexion/extension	146 degrees/WNL	
142 degrees/WNL	Shoulder abd/add	160 degrees/WNL	
WNL	Shoulder IR/ER	WNL	
WNL	Shoulder horizontal abd/add	WNL	
WNL	Elbow flexion/extension	WNL	
WNL	Forearm pronation/supination	WNL	
WNL	Wrist flexion/extension	WNL	

Left	Joint/Joint Complexes	Right	Comments
	Table 2-4 continued		
WNL	MCP flexion/extension	WNL	
WNL	PIP flexion/extension	WNL	
WNL	DIP flexion/extension	WNL	
WNL	Finger abd/add	WNL	
WNL	Thumb MCP flexion/extension	WNL	
WNL	Thumb ICP flexion/extension	WNL	
WNL	Thumb abd/add	WNL	
WNL	Thumb opposition	WNL	
	Lower Extremities		
50 degrees	SLR	45 degrees	
110/0 degrees	Hip flexion/extension	112/-5 degrees	
35/15 degrees	Hip abd/add	40/15 degrees	
WNL/WNL	Hip IR/ER	WNL/WNL	
100/-5 degrees	Knee flexion/extension	104/-8 degrees	
WNL/0 degrees	Ankle plantar/dorsiflexion	WNL/0 degrees	
WFL/5 degrees	Foot eversion/inversion	WFL/5 degrees	
WFL	Great toe flexion/extension	WFL	
WFL	Toe MTP flexion/extension	WFL	
WFL	Toe IP flexion/extension	WFL	

Mod ↓ = moderate decrease; min ↓ = minimal decrease; abd = abduction; add = adduction; IR = internal rotation; ER = external rotation; MCP = metacarpophalangeal; PIP = proximal interphalangeal; DIP = distal interphalangeal; ICP = intermittent oppression pump; WNL = within normal limits; WFL = within functional limits; SLR = straight leg raise.

- *Toilet: Supervised with minimum assistance with cues for technique. No equipment used presently.*
- *Tub/shower: Minimum assistance with moderate cues with seat.*
- *Car: Minimum assistance with minimum cues for technique.*

10. *Gait:* At this time, patient ambulates without an assistive device with a forward flexed posture at the thoracic spine and hips and a wide base of support. She demonstrates festinating gait and uses furniture for support. She requires minimum assistance on stairs due to decreased LE clearance and depth perception issues whether or not a rail is present.

11. *Functional mobility*: She requires supervision to minimum assistance for all functional mobility at the home and community level. Her ambulation technique of "furniture walking" makes safety a significant issue during function at home.

12. *Self-care*: She requires cues and supervision for task initiation during feeding and grooming. She requires minimum assistance for dressing her lower body and toileting. She is dependent for all fasteners.

13. *Home management*: She is dependent for most home management tasks, although she is able to sit at the kitchen table to fold laundry and stand at the sink to wash and dry dishes, which she insists that she do, as her husband does

all the other tasks. She occasionally tries to dust and "tidy up," however her husband discourages this, as she is at significant risk for loss of balance and falls during these activities.

PATIENT GOALS

1. Independent grooming.
2. Independent lower body dressing.
3. Independent toileting.
4. Independent ambulation on all surfaces without a device.
5. Independent transfers.
6. Independent bed mobility.

EXERCISES FOR THE OT AND PT STUDENT

Case # 5: Frances Littleton

1. Using the Nagi scheme of disability, present the active pathology(ies), impairments, functional limitations, and disabilities for this case.

2. Do you think the patient's goals are realistic? Why or why not? If not, what strategies would you use to help the patient focus on more realistic goals?

3. Write an assessment and plan for the patient case(s) assigned. Include appropriate short-term and long-term goals.

4. Present a thorough plan of care for the case (ie, what specifically would you do with this patient and why?)

5. Design a treatment session lasting 30 minutes for this patient.

6. If both occupational and physical therapy were involved with this patient, what would you see as the role for each discipline to provide an appropriate, comprehensive treatment program? Consider the concepts of cotreatment and expert consultation in your answer.

7. Based upon the pathology that the patient exhibits and the individual impairments and functional limitations, do you think the patient will ever become totally "able" again? If not, which disabilities may remain?

8. What compensatory strategies might you teach the patient in this case?

9. What type(s) of DME (orthotic, prosthetic, or adaptive equipment) might you prescribe and why?

10. What would you propose as an appropriate treatment frequency and length of stay for this patient in your treatment setting? Provide the rationale for your answer.

11. What modifications would you have to make to the plan of care if you received insurance approval for only one-half of the time requested and the patient did not want to fund therapy privately?

12. Which portion(s) of the plan of care would you delegate to an assistant? Which portion(s) to an aide/tech? Provide your rationale for your answer.

13. For physical therapy students: Using the *Guidelines for Practice*, what would be your physical therapy diagnosis for this patient?

14. What environment(s) would you choose for implementing your treatment activities?

15. What activities would you use to address this patient's values?

16. Who is this patient? What roles and activities are important to her?

EXERCISES FOR THE ASSISTANT STUDENT

Case #5: Frances Littleton

1. Using the Nagi scheme of disability, present the active pathology(ies), impairments, functional limitations, and disabilities for this case.

2. Design a treatment session lasting 30 minutes for this patient.

3. If both occupational and physical therapy were involved with this patient, what would you see as the role for each discipline to provide an appropriate, comprehensive treatment program? Consider the concepts of cotreatment and expert consultation in your answer.

4. Based upon the pathology that the patient exhibits and the individual impairments and functional limitations, do you think the patient will ever become totally "able" again? If not, which disabilities may remain?

5. What compensatory strategies might you teach the patient in this case?

6. What type(s) of DME (orthotic, prosthetic, or adaptive equipment) might you prescribe and why?

7. Which portion(s) of the plan of care would you delegate to an aide/tech? Provide your rationale for your answer.

8. What environment(s) would you choose for implementing your treatment activities?

9. What activities would you use to address this patient's values?

10. Who is this patient? What roles and activities are important to her?

Right-Middle Cerebrovascular Accident

Marcia Hollis is a 33-year-old woman who, after a divorce from her husband last year, has been the head of a household consisting of her 8-year-old son and her 68-year-old mother.

Since the divorce, no one in the family has seen or heard from her former husband, so Marcia has been responsible for the financial, as well as physical and emotional support of her son. This has been difficult, as last year she was laid off from her job as an administrative assistant and now works as a salesperson in a clothing store. This job provides her with only 75% of her former salary, and she also works 10 hours each week as a waitress in a local family restaurant to supplement her income.

Her mother is quite independent and provides after-school child care for the patient's son. They are a very close-knit family and, until this point, have managed to cope with the changes in their lives fairly well. Marcia, however, has been placed under a great deal of emotional and physical stress due to the changes in her life over the past year.

The family lives in a three-bedroom apartment on one level. There are no architectural barriers once inside the home. The home is entered by four steps without rails leading to the front door. The back door has six steps with a rail. They have lived here for the past year and enjoy the apartment and their neighbors next door, a young couple whom they get together with for dinner every other week.

Last month, Marcia became ill at church and was rushed to the emergency room (ER) and diagnosed with a right middle cerebral artery cerebrovascular accident (CVA). She was admitted to the acute care hospital, then discharged to a rehabilitation hospital 6 days later, where she had 3 weeks of intensive rehabilitation services. She returned home and is discharged to your outpatient center 25 days later for services to regain maximum function.

She presents to you in the clinic with the following findings:
1. *Significant past medical history*: Insulin-dependent diabetes mellitus (IDDM) and HTN. She is a non-smoker. She drinks three to four glasses of wine per week with dinner.
2. *Medications*: NPH and regular insulin, as well as tenormin (Astra Zeneca, Wilmington, Del).
3. *Cognition/perception*: She demonstrates homonymous hemianopsia.

Cognition:
- *Alert and oriented x 3 with environmental cues (ie, calendar)*
- *Attention: Sustained attention but is easily distracted by other sensory stimuli.*
- *Concentration: Minimum to moderate difficulty with sustained concentration.*
- *Memory: WFL*
- *Sequencing: WFL for familiar/functional tasks. Minimum to moderate difficulties with new/unfamiliar tasks.*
- *Ability to follow directions: WFL for verbal and written direction in a quiet environment. Minimum assistance in a distractible environment.*
- *Initiation: WNL*
- *Insight/judgment: WFL.*

- *Problem solving: WFL for basic tasks such as changing a schedule when a problem arises or for basic safety issues at home.*
4. *ROM*: WNL for all extremities and trunk. A small left glenohumeral subluxation is noted.
5. *Strength*: See Table 2-5.

Essentially, there is no active movement in the left upper extremity muscles, but the patient is able to attain full hip flexion with knee flexion and dorsiflexion in supine. Unable to isolate hip external rotation (ER) or internal rotation (IR) on the left LE. Left LE abduction and adduction are through the full range in supine. Isolated hip, knee, or ankle movement is very limited on the left.

6. *Neurological*: Balance is fair in sitting, with the patient being able to reach through minimal excursions during functional tasks. Balance in standing is fair, when wearing left ankle/foot orthosis (AFO) and standing with a small based quad cane (SBQC), able to attain standing with supervision, able to maintain standing and take moderate pushes, and she can move through moderate active trunk excursion with minimum assistance. Sensation is severely impaired with zero out of 10 correct responses for testing of proprioception, light touch, pain, and deep pressure, as well as hot/cold in the left extremities. Tone is moderately impaired with hypotonicity throughout the left lower and upper extremities. Trunk tone is minimally hypotonic. Clonus is noted at the left ankle. Equilibrium reactions and protective extension are moderately impaired in standing and minimally impaired on the left in sitting.

7. *Pain*: Without complaints of pain in any region.
8. *Skin/edema*: Without issue. Patient wears TED stocking as an edema prevention measure.

9. *Mobility*

Bed mobility:
- *Patient is independent in bed mobility without a device.*

Transfers:
- *Sit → stand: Independent with SBQC.*
- *Bed ↔ w/c: Supervised secondary to occasional loss of balance.*
- *Chair ↔ w/c: Supervised secondary to occasional loss of balance.*
- *Toilet: Supervised secondary to occasional loss of balance.*
- *Tub/shower: Minimum assistance with moderate cues with seat.*
- *Car: Minimum assistance with minimum cues for technique.*

10. *Gait*: She is ambulatory, requiring minimum to moderate assistance for balance and LLE control. She uses a SBQC and an AFO for ankle and knee support. She has difficulty with left lower extremity placement and often adducts

Table 2-5

Manual Muscle Test

Left	Muscle/Muscle Group	Right	Comments
Neck			
G	Flexion/extension	G	
G	Rotation	G	
G	Lateral flexion	G	
Trunk			
F	Flexion/extension	F	
F	Rotation	F	
F	Lateral flexion	F	
F	Pelvic elevation	F	
Upper Extremities			
W/o active movement	Scapular abd/add	WNL	
W/o active movement	Scapular elevation	WNL	
W/o active movement	Shoulder flexion/extension	WNL	
W/o active movement	Shoulder abd/add	WNL	
W/o active movement	Shoulder IR/ER	WNL	
W/o active movement	Shoulder horizontal abd/add	WNL	
W/o active movement	Elbow flexion/extension	WNL	
W/o active movement	Forearm pronation/supination	WNL	
W/o active movement	Wrist flexion/extension	WNL	
W/o active movement	MCP flexion/extension	WNL	
W/o active movement	PIP flexion/extension	WNL	
W/o active movement	DIP flexion/extension	WNL	
W/o active movement	Finger abd/add	WNL	
W/o active movement	Thumb MCP flexion/extension	WNL	
W/o active movement	Thumb ICP flexion/extension	WNL	
W/o active movement	Thumb abd/add	WNL	
W/o active movement	Thumb opposition	WNL	
Lower Extremities			
Full AROM in flexor synergy	Hip flexion/extension	WNL	
Full AROM in flexor synergy	Hip abd/add	WNL	
full AROM in flexor synergy	Hip IR/ER	WNL	

Table 2-5 continued

Left	Muscle/Muscle Group	Right	Comments
Full AROM in flexor synergy	Knee flexion/extension	WNL	
Full AROM in flexor synergy	Ankle plantar/dorsiflexion	WNL	
Full AROM in flexor synergy	Foot eversion/inversion	WNL	
W/o isolated movement	Great toe flexion/extension	WNL	
W/o isolated movement	Toe MTP flexion/extension	WNL	
W/o isolated movement	Toe IP flexion/extension	WNL	

abd = abduction; add = adduction; IR = internal rotation; ER = external rotation; MCP = metacarpophalangeal; PIP = proximal interphalangeal; DIP = distal interphalangeal; ICP = intermittent compression pump; WNL = within normal limits.

prior to ground contact, decreasing her base of support and resulting in a loss of balance. She can ambulate 200 feet. She can ascend and descend stairs with a rail using her SBQC and AFO with minimum assistance.

11. *Functional mobility*: She is independent in wheelchair mobility for home-level function. Fortunately, her home accommodates wheelchair use with only the need to move some furniture in the family room to allow the patient to be independent.

12. *Self-care*: She is independent in feeding after set-up. Independent in unilateral grooming tasks but needs maximum assistance for bilateral tasks. She requires minimum assistance for stand-hike for underwear and pants but is otherwise independent. She requires minimum to maximum assistance for toileting. She is dependent for all fasteners.

13. *Home management*: She is able to do light housework tasks such as basic meal preparation with adaptive equipment and dusting independently from a wheelchair level, which she states "makes me feel useful, as I can't work." Her mother is the primary caretaker of the apartment, which was the patient's role prior to her CVA.

PATIENT GOALS

1. Independent bed mobility.
2. Independent transfers.
3. Independent self-care with equipment.
4. Independent ambulation without a device.
5. Minimum assistance in home management.
6. Return to work (patient is willing to work with vocational counselors to alter job type if necessary).

EXERCISES FOR THE OT AND PT STUDENT

Case #6: Marcia Hollis

1. Using the Nagi scheme of disability, present the active pathology(ies), impairments, functional limitations, and disabilities for this case.

2. Do you think the patient's goals are realistic? Why or why not? If not, what strategies would you use to help the patient focus on more realistic goals?

3. Write an assessment and plan for the patient case(s) assigned. Include appropriate short-term and long-term goals.

4. Present a thorough plan of care for the case (ie, what specifically would you do with this patient and why?)

5. Design a treatment session lasting 30 minutes for this patient.

6. If both occupational and physical therapy were involved with this patient, what would you see as the role for each discipline to provide an appropriate, comprehensive treatment program? Consider the concepts of cotreatment and expert consultation in your answer.

7. Based upon the pathology that the patient exhibits and the individual impairments and functional limitations, do you think the patient will ever become totally "able" again? If not, which disabilities may remain?

8. What compensatory strategies might you teach the patient in this case?

9. What type(s) of DME (orthotic, prosthetic, or adaptive equipment) might you prescribe and why?

10. What would you propose as an appropriate treatment frequency and length of stay for this patient in your treatment setting? Provide the rationale for your answer.

11. What modifications would you have to make to the plan of care if you received insurance approval for only one-half of the time requested and the patient did not want to fund therapy privately?

12. Which portion(s) of the plan of care would you delegate to an assistant? Which portion(s) to an aide/tech? Provide your rationale for your answer.

13. For physical therapy students: Using the *Guidelines for Practice*, what would be your physical therapy diagnosis for this patient?

14. What environment(s) would you choose for implementing your treatment activities?

15. What activities would you use to address this patient's values?

16. Who is this patient? What roles and activities are important to her?

EXERCISES FOR THE ASSISTANT STUDENT

Case #6: Marcia Hollis

1. Using the Nagi scheme of disability, present the active pathology(ies), impairments, functional limitations, and disabilities for this case.

2. Design a treatment session lasting 30 minutes for this patient.

3. If both occupational and physical therapy were involved with this patient, what would you see as the role for each discipline to provide an appropriate, comprehensive treatment program? Consider the concepts of cotreatment and expert consultation in your answer.

4. Based upon the pathology that the patient exhibits and the individual impairments and functional limitations, do you think the patient will ever become totally "able" again? If not, which disabilities may remain?

5. What compensatory strategies might you teach the patient in this case?

6. What type(s) of DME (orthotic, prosthetic, or adaptive equipment) might you prescribe and why?

7. Which portion(s) of the plan of care would you delegate to an aide/tech? Provide your rationale for your answer.

8. What environment(s) would you choose for implementing your treatment activities?

9. What activities would you use to address this patient's values?

10. Who is this patient? What roles and activities are important to her?

Left Cerebrovascular Accident

Josephine Tyler is a 78-year-old widow who lives in a "mother-in-law" apartment off her son's new home. There are no steps to enter the apartment and no architectural barriers once inside. She has a stall shower with a built-in seat. She receives assistance with her grocery shopping and cleaning from her son's family. Otherwise, she is independent for all functional activities. She has decorated her apartment with many of her treasures that she has collected over the years. In her younger days, she enjoyed all types of needlecrafts, especially hooking rugs and needlepoint. Her home is a showpiece for many of her works.

Mrs. Tyler has taken good care of herself. Her medical history is significant for CHF, atrial fibrillation (A.-fib), HTN, and osteoporosis for 15 years. She has five adult children and is s/p an appendectomy about 60 years ago. She takes lopressor qd, lasix bid, and Tums with calcium qd.

She supports her lifestyle with social security and her pension, which she receives from her work as a telephone operator. She is a homebody except for Mondays and Wednesdays when she drives to the local senior citizen center. There she participates in a needlework class and enjoys the "stretch and tone" class.

One evening while making dinner, Mrs. Tyler fell in her kitchen. Her daughter-in-law heard the smashing of dishes and raced into the apartment. Mrs. Tyler was rushed to the local emergency room where she was diagnosed with a left middle cerebral artery CVA. After a 7-day acute hospitalization, she is transferred to your facility with orders for evaluation and treatment to regain maximum functional abilities. Mrs. Tyler and her family would like her to return home. The family states that they are willing and able to care for all home management tasks.

The results of the initial evaluation are as follows:

1. *Perception*: Mrs. Tyler wears glasses. Otherwise her perception appears WFL.

2. *Communication*: She has expressive aphasia. She is able to make her needs known approximately 75% of the time using pictorial representation or pantomime.

3. *Cognition*:
   - *Alert and oriented x 3 (appears intact): Is cooperative and active participant; recognizes family members.*
   - *Attention: Attentive during all activities.*
   - *Concentration: Appears WFL.*
   - *Memory: Unable to assess.*
   - *Sequencing: Demonstrates the ability to follow three steps during self feeding and transfers.*
   - *Ability to follow directions: Will mime concrete tasks (ie, transfers).*
   - *Initiation: Appropriate.*
   - *Insight/judgment: Appears intact.*
   - *Problem solving: Appears intact for rote tasks seen during initial visit.*

4. *AROM*: WFL except right trunk has one-half ROM in all planes. There is no AROM of the right upper extremity (RUE) except for shoulder elevation. The RLE has one-half to three-quarters AROM of all hip and knee movements against gravity. Full AROM of RLE without tonal influence in gravity eliminated positioning.

5. *Neurology*: Hypotonicity noted of RUE and right trunk. RLE has minimum to moderate hypotonicity. There is no clonus present.

6. *Sensation/pain*: Sensation is severely impaired with two out 10 correct responses for light touch, pain, proprioception, and deep pressure throughout the right side. She has significant pain of the right glenohumeral (G-H) joint. She rates the pain as a 3 at rest and as a 7 during mobility on a 1 to 10 scale. Sensation on the trunk and the left side is WFL.

7. *Skin/edema*: Intact skin integrity. Moderate distal RLE edema. TED stockings are worn.

8. *Balance*
   - *Static, unsupported sit is F+*
   - *Dynamic sit is P+*
   - *Static stand is P+*
   - *Dynamic stand for minimal excursion is P*

9. *Mobility*

Bed mobility:
   - *Rolling: Onto left side with maximum assistance. Onto right side with moderate assistance.*
   - *Bridging: Maximum assistance with moderate cues.*
   - *Supine ↔ sit: Moderate assistance with moderate cues from the left side.*
   - *Equipment: Half-rails.*

Transfers:
   - *Sit → stand: Moderate assistance for balance and support.*
   - *Bed ↔ wheelchair: Maximum assistance x 1 for stand-step-turn.*
   - *Chair ↔ wheelchair: Maximum assistance x 1 for stand pivot.*
   - *Toilet ↔ wheelchair: Maximum assistance x 1 for squat pivot.*
   - *Tub/shower ↔ wheelchair: Maximum assistance.*
   - *Car: NT.*

10. *Wheelchair mobility*: Moderate assistance primarily for cue for propulsion and maneuvering. She can propel the chair for 50 feet then becomes SOB. Patient requires moderate assistance for locking brakes prior to standing. She requires maximum assistance for leg rest placement and maneuvering.

11. *Gait/functional mobility*: Patient is nonambulatory at present.

12. *Self-care (left dominant):*

   - *Feeding/equipment: She is on a modified diet and is able to self-feed with moderate cues for pocketing.*
   - *Bathing: She bathes seated, sink level with maximum assistance for both upper and lower body tasks. She needs assistance in placing her RUE for support and is unable to bathe her LUE. Stand/wash is also maximum assistance due to balance issues. She is dependent for bathing below her knees and for bed-level bathing.*
   - *Grooming: Once set-up, she is able to comb her hair and wash her face. Oral hygiene is dependent for all set-up, and she brushes her teeth with moderate assistance.*
   - *Dressing: She dresses her upper body with maximum assistance and is dependent for her lower body. RUE and trunk balance hinders her independence.*
   - *Toileting: Maximum assistance for clothing management and hygiene. Is able to lateral weight shift. Some accidents evident due to urgency.*
   - *Home management: NT.*
   - *Leisure/community: To be evaluated at a later time.*

13. *ROM*: See Table 2-6.

14. *Strength*: See Table 2-7.

PATIENT GOALS

1. To return home. Family states they are willing and able to care for all home management tasks.
2. Independent self-feeding.
3. Independent self-care.
4. Independent toileting.
5. Independent transfers, including showering.
6. Independent ambulation with assistive device, if necessary.
7. Return to social activities with minimal assistance/supervision.
8. Return to driving.

EXERCISES FOR THE OT AND PT STUDENT

Case #7: Josephine Tyler

1. Using the Nagi scheme of disability, present the active pathology(ies), impairments, functional limitations, and disabilities for this case.

2. Do you think the patient's goals are realistic? Why or why not? If not, what strategies would you use to help the patient focus on more realistic goals?

3. Write an assessment and plan for the patient case(s) assigned. Include appropriate short-term and long-term goals.

4. Present a thorough plan of care for the case (ie, what specifically would you do with this patient and why?).

Table 2-6

Range of Motion

Left	Joint/Joint Complexes	Right	Comments
	Neck		
WFL	Flexion/extension	WFL	
WFL	Rotation	WFL	
WFL	Lateral flexion	WFL	
	Trunk		
WFL	Flexion/extension	≈ ½ ROM	
WFL	Rotation	≈ ½ ROM	
WFL	Lateral flexion	≈ ½ ROM	
WFL	Pelvic elevation	≈ ½ ROM	
	Upper Extremities		
WFL	Scapular abd/add	WFL	
WFL	Scapular elevation	WFL	
WFL	Shoulder flexion/extension	80/30	Limited by pain, one finger
WFL	Shoulder abd/add	80/0	Subluxation posteriorly
WFL	Shoulder IR/ER	WFL	
WFL	Shoulder horizontal abd/add	N/A	Cannot achieve starting position
WFL	Elbow flexion/extension	WFL	
WFL	Forearm pronation/supination	WFL	
WFL	Wrist flexion/extension	WFL	
WFL	MCP flexion/extension	WFL	
WFL	PIP flexion/extension	WFL	
WFL	DIP flexion/extension	WFL	
WFL	Finger abd/add	WFL	
WFL	Thumb MCP flexion/extension	WFL	
WFL	Thumb ICP flexion/extension	WFL	
WFL	Thumb abd/add	WFL	
WFL	Thumb opposition	WFL	
	Lower Extremities		
WFL	SLR	WFL	
WFL	Hip flexion/extension	WFL	
WFL	Hip abd/add	WFL	

Table 2-6 continued

Left	Joint/Joint Complexes	Right	Comments
WFL	Hip IR/ER	WFL	
WFL	Knee flexion/extension	WFL	
WFL	Ankle plantar/dorsiflexion	45/-5	
WFL	Foot eversion/inversion	WFL	
WFL	Great toe flexion/extension	WFL	
WFL	Toe MTP flexion/extension	WFL	
WFL	Toe IP flexion/extension	WFL	

abd = abduction; add = adduction; IR = internal rotation; ER = external rotation; MCP = metacarpophalangeal; PIP = proximal interphalangeal; DIP = distal interphalangeal; ICP = intermittent compression pump; WFL = within functional limits; WNL = within normal limits; ≈ approximately.

Table 2-7

Manual Muscle Test

Left	Muscle/Muscle Group	Right	Comments
	Neck		
G-	Flexion/extension	F-	
G-	Rotation	F-	
G-	Lateral flexion	F-	
	Trunk		
F+	Flexion/extension	P	
F+	Rotation	P	
F+	Lateral flexion	P	
F+	Pelvic elevation	P	
	Upper Extremities		
G-/N	Scapular abd/add	0	
G-/N	Scapular elevation	F+	
G-/N	Shoulder flexion/extension		NT
G-/N	Shoulder abd/add		NT
G-/N	Shoulder IR/ER		NT
G-/N	Shoulder horizontal abd/add		NT
G-/N	Elbow flexion/extension		NT

Table 2-7 continued

Left	Muscle/Muscle Group	Right	Comments
G-/N	Forearm pronation/supination		NT
G-/N	Wrist flexion/extension		NT
G-/N	MCP flexion/extension		NT
G-/N	PIP flexion/extension		NT
G-/N	DIP flexion/extension		NT
G-/N	Finger abd/add		NT
G-/N	Thumb MCP flexion/extension		NT
G-/N	Thumb ICP flexion/extension		NT
G-/N	Thumb abd/add		NT
G-/N	Thumb opposition		NT
	Lower Extremities		
G-/N	Hip flexion/extension	P	
G-/N	Hip abd/add	P	
G-/N	Hip IR/ER	P	
G-/N	Knee flexion/extension	P	
G-/N	Ankle plantar/dorsiflexion	P	P- for dorsiflexion
G-/N	Foot eversion/inversion	P	
G-/N	Great toe flexion/extension	P	
G-/N	Toe MTP flexion/extension	P	
G-/N	Toe IP flexion/extension	P	

abd = abduction; add = adduction; IR = internal rotation; ER = external rotation; MCP = metacarpophalangeal; PIP = proximal interphalangeal; DIP = distal interphalangeal; ICP = intermittent oppression pump; WNL = within normal limits; WFL = within functional limits; SLR = straight leg raise; G = good (80%); G+ = good (90%); F = fair (50%); F+ = fair (60%); F- = fair (40%); P = poor (20%); P+ = poor (30%); P- = poor (10%).

5. Design a treatment session lasting 30 minutes for this patient.

6. If both occupational and physical therapy were involved with this patient, what would you see as the role for each discipline to provide an appropriate, comprehensive treatment program? Consider the concepts of cotreatment and expert consultation in your answer.

7. Based upon the pathology that the patient exhibits and the individual impairments and functional limitations, do you think the patient will ever become totally "able" again? If not, which disabilities may remain?

8. What compensatory strategies might you teach the patient in this case?

9. What type(s) of DME (orthotic, prosthetic, or adaptive equipment) might you prescribe and why?

10. What would you propose as an appropriate treatment frequency and length of stay for this patient in your treatment setting? Provide the rationale for your answer.

11. What modifications would you have to make to the plan of care if you received insurance approval for only one-half of the time requested and the patient did not want to fund therapy privately?

12. Which portion(s) of the plan of care would you delegate to an assistant? Which portion(s) to an aide/tech? Provide your rationale for your answer.

13. For physical therapy students: Using the *Guidelines for Practice*, what would be your physical therapy diagnosis for this patient?

14. What environment(s) would you choose for implementing your treatment activities?

15. What activities would you use to address this patient's values?

16. Who is this patient? What roles and activities are important to her?

EXERCISES FOR THE ASSISTANT STUDENT

Case #7: Josephine Tyler

1. Using the Nagi scheme of disability, present the active pathology(ies), impairments, functional limitations, and disabilities for this case.

2. Design a treatment session lasting 30 minutes for this patient.

3. If both occupational and physical therapy were involved with this patient, what would you see as the role for each discipline to provide an appropriate, comprehensive treatment program? Consider the concepts of cotreatment and expert consultation in your answer.

4. Based upon the pathology that the patient exhibits and the individual impairments and functional limitations, do you think the patient will ever become totally "able" again? If not, which disabilities may remain?

5. What compensatory strategies might you teach the patient in this case?

6. What type(s) of DME (orthotic, prosthetic, or adaptive equipment) might you prescribe and why?

7. Which portion(s) of the plan of care would you delegate to an aide/tech? Provide your rationale for your answer.

8. What environment(s) would you choose for implementing your treatment activities?

9. What activities would you use to address this patient's values?

10. Who is this patient? What roles and activities are important to her?

Multiple Sclerosis: Barbara Lighting

Barbara Lighting is a gregarious divorced woman in her late 50s with a 30-year history of multiple sclerosis. She has an adult son who lives on his own in a neighboring town. He has weekly contact with his mother, but his schedule does not allow him to visit regularly. While her son was growing up, Barbara would have exacerbations, which would affect her strength and mobil-

ity. She would try to keep up with her commitments to run the household and make everything seem as normal as possible. Her husband, an ambitious lawyer, was not available to assist her at home. Barbara states the marriage was over when he finally realized that she was not able to "fit the bill" of being a successful lawyer's wife. Many times she was too tired to attend social engagements. She reports that they went on as a couple until he finally lost it and accused her of being tired to avoid social obligations. After a bitter separation and divorce, she moved into a street-level apartment with ramped access.

She has taken only a few choice pieces from her home and decided to start anew. Although ramped, the apartment is not considered handicapped accessible. It has a standard bathroom, but management installed three horizontal grab bars in the tub area and one next to the toilet. The hallway is narrow and the kitchen is galley-style. She spends her mornings sitting in the kitchen. Several times, she has nearly fallen because she has missed her chair. All the chairs are on wheels. In the afternoons, she rests, keeping her portable phone with her at all times. She is seen using her rolling walker while carrying her phone in her hand. Due to her recent exacerbation, Barbara is quite homebound. Both lower extremities are weak with impaired sensation. Right foot drop is evident. Her sit to stand and all transfers are impeded by her loss of balance, especially into the tub area. She dresses sitting on a swivel chair. Her other options include sitting on the edge of the bed or in a rocking chair. After walking approximately 30 feet, fatigue and safety concerns become more visible. She relies on friends to bring her groceries, but she is reluctant to ask. Her son assists with the laundry, but he cannot be counted on.

Barbara is referred to your home health agency upon discharge from her recent acute hospitalization. She had received therapy services in the past while living with her husband. Her goals are to remain independent in the community. She realistically states she is unable to carry her groceries into the apartment, nor is she able to access the laundry room. She plans to resume driving when she is able and reports being on a fixed income because her support from her ex-spouse is unreliable.

The results of her initial evaluation are as follows:

1. *Cognition/perception*: She has a right visual field cut that interferes with her peripheral vision. She reports that during exacerbations she has diplopia.

Cognition:

- *Alert and oriented x 3*
- *Attention: WFL. Can maintain vigilance but deteriorates with distraction.*
- *Concentration: WFL for sustained tasks but impaired divided concentration.*
- *Memory: Overall, WFL. Difficulty sometimes seen with immediate recall, especially for new data.*
- *Sequencing: WNL*
- *Ability to follow directions: WFL.*
- *Initiation: Can be impulsive*

- *Insight/judgment: Fair. At times, she does not incorporate safe techniques (ie, carrying phone in hand while using her walker). She can also appear euphoric.*
- *Problem solving: Can generate appropriate solutions but does not incorporate them into function. Also, recognizes that home management is an issue but does not act to solve.*

2. *Motor control*: Trunk has diminished tone with mild ataxic gait.

3. *Sensation/pain*: Paresthesia and impaired position sense noted of bilateral lower extremities (BLE). Ms. Lighting has no complaints of pain.

4. *Skin/edema*: Essentially unremarkable.

5. *Balance*: Patient maintains good static supported sitting. However, she easily loses her balance at the edge of the bed. This loss of balance is exaggerated during any excursions (dressing lower body). Static stand with walker is F+ with center of gravity easily shifted with challenges.

6. *Mobility*

Bed Mobility:
- *Rolling: Independent—patient pulls on side of mattress to achieve side lying.*
- *Bridging: Independent.*
- *Supine ↔ sit: Poor control—several attempts to achieve it. Patient states that it sometimes takes her 20 minutes.*
- *Equipment: None.*

Transfers:
- *Sit → stand: Independent in straight chair with armrests (impaired safety with loss of balance).*
- *Bed ↔ rolling walker: Independent to moderate assistance (difficulty achieving anterior pelvic tilt).*
- *Chair ↔ rolling walker: Minimum assistance from rocker or a swivel chair with loss of balance.*
- *Toilet ↔ rolling walker: Independent with use of grab bars.*
- *Tub/shower ↔ tub seat, grab bars, and rolling walker: Loss of balance at minimum assistance.*
- *Car: NT.*

7. *Gait/functional mobility*: Ms. Lighting uses a rolling walker at all times. She is a safety risk secondary to her lower extremity function and sensation issues. She is observed walking with the walker handle and phone in her hand at the same time. Right foot drop is evident with area rugs in the main rooms placed over wall-to-wall carpeting. At times, she will brace herself on stable surfaces to obtain items from storage.

8. *Self-care*
- *Feeding/equipment: Independent. Eats balanced simple meals.*

- *Bathing: Seated, she is able to bathe all body parts and performs a lateral weight shift for pericare.*
- *Grooming: Uses good upper extremity stabilization techniques. Has a no-fuss short hairstyle.*
- *Dressing: Labor-intensive task. Dresses sitting on a swivel chair that displaces her center of gravity when she performs lower body tasks. Sit to stand is unsafe due to fatigue.*
- *Toileting: Performs independently but reports bouts of urinary incontinence, which makes clothing management and hygiene difficult.*
- *Home management: Completes light meal preparation daily (toast, soup, frozen dinners). Relies on others for laundry, shopping, and cleaning.*
- *Leisure/community: Is in touch with the world through her portable phone. Currently is homebound. Friends plan to drive her to any appointments that she may have.*

9. *ROM*: See Table 2-8.

10. *Strength*: See Table 2-9.

PATIENT GOALS

1. Independent showering.
2. Independent, safe dressing.
3. Independent ambulation in home without fear of falling.
4. Independent transfers to all surfaces.
5. A regular plan for home management tasks.
6. To return to the community and driving when possible.

EXERCISES FOR THE OT AND PT STUDENT

Case #8: Barbara Lighting

1. Using the Nagi scheme of disability, present the active pathology(ies), impairments, functional limitations, and disabilities for this case.

2. Do you think the patient's goals are realistic? Why or why not? If not, what strategies would you use to help the patient focus on more realistic goals?

3. Write an assessment and plan for the patient case(s) assigned. Include appropriate short-term and long-term goals.

4. Present a thorough plan of care for the case (ie, what specifically would you do with this patient and why?)

5. Design a treatment session lasting 30 minutes for this patient.

6. If both occupational and physical therapy were involved with this patient, what would you see as the role for each discipline to provide an appropriate, comprehensive treatment program? Consider the concepts of cotreatment and expert consultation in your answer.

<u>Table 2-8</u>
Range of Motion

Left	Joint/Joint Complexes	Right	Comments
	Neck		
WFL	Flexion/extension	WFL	
WFL	Rotation	WFL	
WFL	Lateral flexion	WFL	
	Trunk		
WFL	Flexion/extension	WFL	
WFL	Rotation	WFL	
WFL	Lateral flexion	WFL	
WFL	Pelvic elevation	WFL	
	Upper Extremities		
WFL	Scapular abd/add	WFL	
WFL	Scapular elevation	WFL	
WFL	Shoulder flexion/extension	WFL	
WFL	Shoulder abd/add	WFL	
WFL	Shoulder IR/ER	WFL	
WFL	Shoulder horizontal abd/add	WFL	
WFL	Elbow flexion/extension	WFL	
WFL	Forearm pronation/supination	WFL	
WFL	Wrist flexion/extension	WFL	
WFL	MCP flexion/extension	WFL	
WFL	PIP flexion/extension	WFL	
WFL	DIP flexion/extension	WFL	
WFL	Finger abd/add	WFL	
WFL	Thumb MCP flexion/extension	WFL	
WFL	Thumb ICP flexion/extension	WFL	
WFL	Thumb abd/add	WFL	
WFL	Thumb opposition	WFL	
	Lower Extremities		
WFL	SLR	WFL	
WFL	Hip flexion/extension	WFL	
WFL	Hip abd/add	WFL	

<u>Table 2-8 continued</u>

Left	Joint/Joint Complexes	Right	Comments
WFL	Hip IR/ER	WFL	
WFL	Knee flexion/extension	WFL	
WFL	Ankle plantar/dorsiflexion	WFL	
WFL	Foot eversion/inversion	WFL	
WFL	Great toe flexion/extension	WFL	
WFL	Toe MTP flexion/extension	WFL	
WFL	Toe IP flexion/extension	WFL	

abd = abduction; add = adduction; IR = internal rotation; ER = external rotation; MCP = metacarpophalangeal; PIP = proximal interphalangeal; DIP = distal interphalangeal; ICP = intermittent oppression pump; WFL = within functional limits.

<u>Table 2-9</u>

Manual Muscle Test

Left	Muscle/Muscle Group	Right	Comments
	Neck		
G/G-	Flexion/extension	G/G-	
G/G-	Rotation	G/G-	
G/G-	Lateral flexion	G/G-	
	Trunk		
G-/F+	Flexion/extension	G-/F+	
G-/F+	Rotation	G-/F+	
G-/F+	Lateral flexion	G-/F+	
G-/F+	Pelvic elevation	G-/F+	
	Upper Extremities		
G-/G	Scapular abd/add	G	
G-/G	Scapular elevation	G	
G-/G	Shoulder flexion/extension	G	
G-/G	Shoulder abd/add	G	
G-/G	Shoulder IR/ER	G	
G-/G	Shoulder horizontal abd/add	G	

Table 2-9 continued

Left	Muscle/Muscle Group	Right	Comments
N	Elbow flexion/extension	N	
G+	Forearm pronation/supination	G+	
G	Wrist flexion/extension	G+	
G	MCP flexion/extension	G+	
G	PIP flexion/extension	G+	
G	DIP flexion/extension	G+	
G	Finger abd/add	G+	
G	Thumb MCP flexion/extension	G+	
G	Thumb ICP flexion/extension	G+	
G	Thumb abd/add	G+	
G	Thumb opposition	G+	
	Lower Extremities		
G	Hip flexion/extension	G-	
G-/G	Hip abd/add	G-	
G/G-	Hip IR/ER	G-/F+	
F+/G-	Knee flexion/extension	F+/G-	
F+/G-	Ankle plantar/dorsiflexion	P+	
F+/G-	Foot eversion/inversion	P+	
F+/G-	Great toe flexion/extension	P+	
F+/G-	Toe MTP flexion/extension	P+	
F+/G-	Toe IP flexion/extension	P+	

abd = abduction; add = adduction; IR = internal rotation; ER = external rotation; MCP = metacarpophalangeal; PIP = proximal interphalangeal; DIP = distal interphalangeal; ICP = intermittent compression pump; WNL = within normal limits; WFL = within functional limits; SLR = straight leg raise; G = good (80%); G+ = good (90%); F = fair (50%); F+ = fair (60%); F- = fair (40%); P = poor (20%); P+ = poor (30%); P- = poor (10%).

7. Based upon the pathology that the patient exhibits and the individual impairments and functional limitations, do you think the patient will ever become totally "able" again? If not, which disabilities may remain?

8. What compensatory strategies might you teach the patient in this case?

9. What type(s) of DME (orthotic, prosthetic, or adaptive equipment) might you prescribe and why?

10. What would you propose as an appropriate treatment frequency and length of stay for this patient in your treatment setting? Provide the rationale for your answer.

11. What modifications would you have to make to the plan of care if you received insurance approval for only one-half of the time requested and the patient did not want to fund therapy privately?

12. Which portion(s) of the plan of care would you delegate to an assistant? Which portion(s) to an aide/tech? Provide your rationale for your answer.

13. For physical therapy students: Using the *Guidelines for Practice*, what would be your physical therapy diagnosis for this patient?

14. What environment(s) would you choose for implementing your treatment activities?

15. What activities would you use to address this patient's values?

16. Who is this patient? What roles and activities are important to her?

EXERCISES FOR THE ASSISTANT STUDENT

Case #8: Barbara Lighting

1. Using the Nagi scheme of disability, present the active pathology(ies), impairments, functional limitations, and disabilities for this case.

2. Design a treatment session lasting 30 minutes for this patient.

3. If both occupational and physical therapy were involved with this patient, what would you see as the role for each discipline to provide an appropriate, comprehensive treatment program? Consider the concepts of cotreatment and expert consultation in your answer.

4. Based upon the pathology that the patient exhibits and the individual impairments and functional limitations, do you think the patient will ever become totally "able" again? If not, which disabilities may remain?

5. What compensatory strategies might you teach the patient in this case?

6. What type(s) of DME (orthotic, prosthetic, or adaptive equipment) might you prescribe and why?

7. Which portion(s) of the plan of care would you delegate to an aide/tech? Provide your rationale for your answer.

8. What environment(s) would you choose for implementing your treatment activities?

9. What activities would you use to address this patient's values?

10. Who is this patient? What roles and activities are important to her?

Multiple Sclerosis: Janice Smithfield

Janice Smithfield is a 41-year-old energetic, career-oriented single woman who is the CEO of a large health care corporation. She devotes 60 to 70 hours per week to her vocation, but in her leisure time enjoys aerobic dancing three to five times per week, attending the ballet, and taking conversational Spanish classes in the evening. She has many friends in the immediate geographical area and enjoys an active social life. Despite the hectic pace of her career, she is known as a friend who is there when you need her. Her family consists of her mother and father as well as two sisters and a brother, all of whom live at least a 2-hour plane flight away. Janice is able to visit with each of them at least once a year, as her business trips are frequent and often to locations near one of their residences.

Two months ago, Janice began having episodes of diplopia. At first she disregarded them as due to fatigue and jet lag, but she later went for an eye examination. At the time of the visit and for the week prior, she did not have any episodes of diplopia. The opthalmologist's examination was normal but she did tell Janice that if the diplopia returned, she should consult a neurologist to make sure that there was nothing neurological causing this disturbance. Shortly after this visit, Janice began having frequent episodes of numbness and tingling in her hands and feet. She also noticed prolonged fatigue after her aerobics workout and, in fact, had occasionally caught her right foot and stumbled during aerobics or when climbing stairs. Janice became concerned and made an appointment with a neurologist for consultation.

At the time of the consultation, the neurologist stated that her clinical signs and symptoms made it possible that Janice had multiple sclerosis. She became alarmed but was able to control her emotions and agreed to have an MRI to confirm the diagnosis. The results of the MRI confirmed multiple sclerosis. Her neurologist stated that her symptoms appear to indicate a progressive form of MS with possible exacerbating-remitting signs and symptoms. Janice immediately wanted to find out more about the disease and how to cope with it. The neurologist suggested that she contact the Multiple Sclerosis Foundation for information and support, and that she have some rehabilitative services to maximize her functional abilities. Janice wholeheartedly agreed and stated that she would do whatever it took to maintain her lifestyle. She is now referred to your outpatient clinic for treatment.

She presents to you in the clinic with the following findings:

1. *Significant past medical history*: Without significant PMH.

2. *Medications*: Ibuprofen.

3. *Cognition/perception*: WNL for cognition and perception. Vision is WNL unless she is having an episode of diplopia. These episodes render her unable to read or drive and make functional mobility at an ambulatory level difficult. A typical episode lasts 1 to 2 hours.

4. *Sensation*: Intact for all sensory modalities with complaints of painful sensory disturbance throughout her RUE and occasionally in her distal bilateral lower extremities.

5. *ROM*: WNL throughout.

6. *Strength*: See Table 2-10.

7. *Balance/coordination*: WNL in sitting. In standing, balance is impaired with patient reports of almost falling twice in the last month as her "right leg just went out from under her." She is unable to perform unilateral stance on the RLE for more than 5 seconds. Without deficit in UE coordination but with minimal deficits in LE coordination, primarily on the right noted during tandem walking, braiding, and reciprocal alternating movement tasks.

<u>Table 2-10</u>

Manual Muscle Test

Left	Muscle/Muscle Group	Right	Comments
	Neck		
WNL	Flexion/extension	WNL	
WNL	Rotation	WNL	
WNL	Lateral flexion	WNL	
	Trunk		
WNL	Flexion/extension	WNL	
WNL	Rotation	WNL	
WNL	Lateral flexion	WNL	
WNL	Pelvic elevation	WNL	
	Upper Extremities		
WNL	Scapular abd/add	WNL	
WNL	Scapular elevation	WNL	
WNL	Shoulder flexion/extension	WNL	
WNL	Shoulder abd/add	WNL	
WNL	Shoulder IR/ER	WNL	
WNL	Shoulder horizontal abd/add	WNL	
WNL	Elbow flexion/extension	WNL	
WNL	Forearm pronation/supination	WNL	
WNL	Wrist flexion/extension	WNL	
WNL	MCP flexion/extension	WNL	
WNL	PIP flexion/extension	WNL	
WNL	DIP flexion/extension	WNL	
WNL	Finger abd/add	WNL	
WNL	Thumb MCP flexion/extension	WNL	
WNL	Thumb ICP flexion/extension	WNL	
WNL	Thumb abd/add	WNL	
WNL	Thumb opposition	WNL	
	Lower Extremities		
WNL	Hip flexion/extension	N/G-	
WNL	Hip abd/add	G/G-	
WNL	Hip IR/ER	G/G	

Left	Muscle/Muscle Group	Right	Comments
WNL	Knee flexion/extension	G/G-	
WNL	Ankle plantar/dorsiflexion	G-/F+	
WNL	Foot eversion/inversion	F+/F+	
WNL	Great toe flexion/extension	F+/F	
WNL	Toe MTP flexion/extension	F+/F	
WNL	Toe IP flexion/extension	F+/F	

abd = abduction; add = adduction; IR = internal rotation; ER = external rotation; MCP = metacarpophalangeal; PIP = proximal interphalangeal; DIP = distal interphalangeal; ICP = intermittent compression pump; WNL = within normal limits; WFL = within functional limits; SLR = straight leg raise; G = good (80%); G+ = good (90%); F = fair (50%); F+ = fair (60%); F- = fair (40%); P = poor (20%); P+ = poor (30%); P- = poor (10%).

8. *Mobility*
   - *Bed mobility: Bed mobility is independent.*
   - *Transfers: Independent for all transfers.*

9. *Gait*: Independent on level, indoor surfaces approximately 95% of the time with the issue of right lower extremity buckling with near falls this past month. Gait analysis reveals poor heel strike to push-off on the right, especially after ambulating on a treadmill at 1.0 mph for 10 minutes due to muscle fatigue, weakness, and poor motor response to changing surfaces such as outdoor, uneven surfaces and stairs without a rail. She can ambulate only 1000 feet without the onset of fatigue. Ambulation on uneven surfaces and stairs without rails requires supervision/occasional minimum assistance due to loss of balance and muscle fatigue, especially in the right tibialis anterior resulting in foot drop.

10. *Functional mobility*: She is independent in all functional mobility most of the time but due to her report of recent right lower extremity weakness with near falls, may benefit from supervision, an orthosis, and/or an assistive device when performing high-level functional mobility tasks such as community ambulation and lifting and carrying objects while ambulatory.

11. *Self-care*: She is independent in all aspects of self-care at this time.

12. *Home management*: She has a housekeeper once a week to complete most household chores and is independent in basic daily home management tasks. She orders her groceries from an online service that delivers to her home one evening each week. She hires individuals to perform all home maintenance projects.

PATIENT GOALS

1. Independent ambulation on all surfaces, preferably without an assistive device.
2. Independent functional mobility at an ambulatory level.
3. Return to regular exercise even if it has to be modified.
4. Maximum conditioning for performance of high physical and mental endurance.

EXERCISES FOR THE OT AND PT STUDENT

Case #12: Janice Smithfield

1. Using the Nagi scheme of disability, present the active pathology(ies), impairments, functional limitations, and disabilities for this case.
2. Do you think the patient's goals are realistic? Why or why not? If not, what strategies would you use to help the patient focus on more realistic goals?
3. Write an assessment and plan for the patient case(s) assigned. Include appropriate short-term and long-term goals.
4. Present a thorough plan of care for the case (ie, what specifically would you do with this patient and why?)
5. Design a treatment session lasting 30 minutes for this patient.
6. If both occupational and physical therapy were involved with this patient, what would you see as the role for each discipline to provide an appropriate, comprehensive treatment program? Consider the concepts of cotreatment and expert consultation in your answer.
7. Based upon the pathology that the patient exhibits and the individual impairments and functional limitations, do you

think the patient will ever become totally "able" again? If not, which disabilities may remain?

8. What compensatory strategies might you teach the patient in this case?

9. What type(s) of DME (orthotic, prosthetic, or adaptive equipment) might you prescribe and why?

10. What would you propose as an appropriate treatment frequency and length of stay for this patient in your treatment setting? Provide the rationale for your answer.

11. What modifications would you have to make to the plan of care if you received insurance approval for only one-half of the time requested and the patient did not want to fund therapy privately?

12. Which portion(s) of the plan of care would you delegate to an assistant? Which portion(s) to an aide/tech? Provide your rationale for your answer.

13. For physical therapy students: Using the *Guidelines for Practice*, what would be your physical therapy diagnosis for this patient?

14. What environment(s) would you choose for implementing your treatment activities?

15. What activities would you use to address this patient's values?

16. Who is this patient? What roles and activities are important to her?

17. How might the stress of her job affect her primary pathology and the resultant impairments and functional limitations?

EXERCISES FOR THE ASSISTANT STUDENT

Case #12: Janice Smithfield

1. Using the Nagi scheme of disability, present the active pathology(ies), impairments, functional limitations, and disabilities for this case.

2. Design a treatment session lasting 30 minutes for this patient.

3. If both occupational and physical therapy were involved with this patient, what would you see as the role for each discipline to provide an appropriate, comprehensive treatment program? Consider the concepts of cotreatment and expert consultation in your answer.

4. Based upon the pathology that the patient exhibits and the individual impairments and functional limitations, do you think the patient will ever become totally "able" again? If not, which disabilities may remain?

5. What compensatory strategies might you teach the patient in this case?

6. What type(s) of DME (orthotic, prosthetic, or adaptive equipment) might you prescribe and why?

7. Which portion(s) of the plan of care would you delegate to an aide/tech? Provide your rationale for your answer.

8. What environment(s) would you choose for implementing your treatment activities?

9. What activities would you use to address this patient's values?

10. Who is this patient? What roles and activities are important to them?

11. How might the stress of her job affect her primary pathology and the resultant impairments and functional limitations?

Amyotrophic Lateral Sclerosis

Martin VanWilkinson was an average 51-year-old man. He was married with two teenaged children—a 14-year-old daughter and a 17-year-old son. He was a house painter who also enjoyed yard work and tackling repairs around his home. Frequently, he had more than one project going on at a time. Martin was active in community soccer by volunteering to coach each season. He was particularly known for his booming voice. Weekly, he would visit with extended family and friends. He was known to enjoy entertaining, especially during the grilling season, as he would try the newest barbecue sauces. His wife was after him to watch his diet, weight, and activity levels. He readily dismissed her concerns. After all, it was not uncommon for a man his age to have HTN and to be overweight. Thirty pounds was not all that much. Also, he felt that he worked hard. He had little need to be involved in any regular fitness program.

Gradually over time, Martin began to have increasing complaints of weakness and stiffness. This progression occurred slowly and it started in his right upper extremity. At times, his hand felt stiff and twitching occurred in his biceps. Martin shrugged off these aches and pains and contributed them to an "overuse" problem that he had heard about on the news. Tylenol prn became a part of his regular regime. Then he noticed he was losing his muscle definition in his right arm. It was at this time that he pursued medical intervention. The diagnosis of Lou Gehrig's disease, or amyotrophic lateral sclerosis (ALS), was devastating. His wife researched everything she could from the local university library. She tried to be supportive and assisted him as necessary. Within months of the diagnosis, all of his extremities became involved, including his head and neck. Eating a meal became a major endeavor. Martin's change in function put stress on his entire family, emotionally and financially.

His family continued to care for Martin at home as long as they were able. As he became dependent for all mobility, they made a family decision to pursue placement for him in a skilled nursing facility. Their hope was for him to receive therapy to get stronger and for them to obtain some respite.

He has treatment orders for evaluation and treatment to regain maximum functional abilities. His goals are to return home to his family and to his social life, including coaching soccer. He would like to feed himself with little assistance and require only physical assistance for bed mobility and transfers.

The results of the initial evaluation are as follows:

1. *Perception/cognition:* WNL

   Cognition:

   - *Alert and oriented x 3*
   - *Attention: WNL*
   - *Concentration: WNL*
   - *Memory: WNL*
   - *Sequencing: WNL*
   - *Ability to follow directions: WNL*
   - *Initiation: WNL*
   - *Insight/judgment: Upon discussion, he is quite aware of his illness and its course. At times, he appears to be unrealistic regarding his capabilities.*
   - *Bed atrophy noted throughout, especially all dorsal interosseous spaces along with impaired breath control while speaking.*

2. *Sensation/pain:* Sensation is intact and there are no complaints of pain.

3. *Skin/edema:* Unremarkable.

4. *Balance:* Unsupported static sit is poor. He can maintain upright with supportive seating. Standing balance is not evaluated.

5. *Mobility*
   - *Rolling: Maximum assistance.*
   - *Bridging: Maximum assistance.*
   - *Supine ↔ sit: Maximum assistance x 2.*
   - *Equipment: Half-rails for rolling.*

   Transfers:
   - *Sit → stand: Dependent.*
   - *Bed ↔ wheelchair: Maximum assistance with slide board.*
   - *Chair ↔ N/A: Likes to sit in recliner with electric controls at home.*
   - *Toilet ↔ drop arm commode: Maximum assistance x 2.*
   - *Tub/shower ↔ wheelchair: Maximum assistance using transfer bench.*
   - *Car: To be evaluated.*

6. *Wheelchair mobility:* Dependent in a manual wheelchair.

7. *Gait/functional mobility:* Dependent.

8. *Self-care:*
   - *Feeding/equipment: Moderate assistance with lightweight, enlarged-handle silverware. Bilateral upper extremities (BUE) are supported on the tabletop. Meal must be set-up. Does better with finger foods. Eats slowly and head/neck becomes increasingly flexed forward as the meal progresses.*
   - *Bathing: Maximum assistance. Bathes upper body, bed level. Able to participate in bathing his lower body by resting one ankle on the other knee. Needs assistance to achieve this position. Dependent for entire backside of body and peri-area.*
   - *Grooming: Maximum assistance. Drops razor and has problems with fatigue and repetitive movements.*
   - *Dressing: Maximum assistance. Wears sweatsuits. Dependent for footwear.*
   - *Toileting: Uses urinal with assistance for set-up. Is on a bowel program. Requires maximum assistance for hygiene and clothing management.*
   - *Home management: Not applicable (NA).*
   - *Leisure/community: Dependent on others for participation.*

9. *ROM:* See Tables 2-11 and 2-12.

10. *Strength:* See Table 2-13.

PATIENT GOALS

1. Minimum assistance and timely self feeding.

2. Maximum assistance for bed mobility in his own bed without rails.

3. Maximum assistance from his spouse for all functional transfers to bed, toilet, recliner, wheelchair, and car.

4. Moderate assistance for toileting and hygiene.

5. Return to social activities with the assistance of family/friends.

6. Return to coaching soccer.

EXERCISES FOR THE OT AND PT STUDENT

Case #9: Martin VanWilkinson

1. Using the Nagi scheme of disability, present the active pathology(ies), impairments, functional limitations, and disabilities for this case.

2. Do you think the patient's goals are realistic? Why or why not? If not, what strategies would you use to help the patient focus on more realistic goals?

3. Write an assessment and plan for the patient case(s) assigned. Include appropriate short-term and long-term goals.

4. Present a thorough plan of care for the case (ie, what specifically would you do with this patient and why?)

5. Design a treatment session lasting 30 minutes for this patient.

Table 2-11
Range of Motion

Left	Joint/Joint Complexes	Right	Comments
	Neck		
WNL	Flexion/extension	WNL	
WNL	Rotation	WNL	
WNL	Lateral flexion	WNL	
	Trunk		
WNL	Flexion/extension	WNL	
WNL	Rotation	WNL	
WNL	Lateral flexion	WNL	
WNL	Pelvic elevation	WNL	
	Upper Extremities		
WNL	Scapular abd/add	WNL	
WNL	Scapular elevation	WNL	
WNL	Shoulder flexion/extension	WNL	
WNL	Shoulder abd/add	WNL	
WNL	Shoulder IR/ER	WNL	
WNL	Shoulder horizontal abd/add	WNL	
WNL	Elbow flexion/extension	WNL	
WNL	Forearm pronation/supination	WNL	
WNL	Wrist flexion/extension	WNL	
WNL	MCP flexion/extension	WNL	
WNL	PIP flexion/extension	WNL	
WNL	DIP flexion/extension	WNL	
WNL	Finger abd/add	WNL	
WNL	Thumb MCP flexion/extension	WNL	
WNL	Thumb ICP flexion/extension	WNL	
WNL	Thumb abd/add	WNL	
WNL	Thumb opposition	WNL	
	Lower Extremities		
WNL	SLR	WNL	
WNL	Hip flexion/extension	WNL	
WNL	Hip abd/add	WNL	

Table 2-11 continued

Left	Joint/Joint Complexes	Right	Comments
WNL	Hip IR/ER	WNL	
WNL	Knee flexion/extension	WNL	
WNL	Ankle plantar/dorsiflexion	WNL	
WNL	Foot eversion/inversion	WNL	
WNL	Great toe flexion/extension	WNL	
WNL	Toe MTP flexion/extension	WNL	
WNL	Toe IP flexion/extension	WNL	

abd = abduction; add = adduction; IR = internal rotation; ER = external rotation; MCP = metacarpophalangeal; PIP = proximal interphalangeal; DIP = distal interphalangeal; ICP = intermittent compression pump; WNL = within normal limits; WFL = within functional limits

Table 2-12

Active Range of Motion

Left	Joint/Joint Complexes	Right	Comments
	Neck		
≈ 3/4	Flexion/extension	≈ 3/4	
≈ 3/4	Rotation	≈ 3/4	
≈ 3/4	Lateral flexion	≈ 3/4	
	Trunk		
≈ 1/4/full	Flexion/extension	≈ 1/4	
≈ 1/4	Rotation	≈ 1/4	
≈ 1/4	Lateral flexion	≈ 1/4	
≈ 1/4	Pelvic elevation	≈ 1/4	
	Upper Extremities		
≈ 1/2	Scapular abd/add	≈ 1/2	
≈ 3/4	Scapular elevation	≈ 3/4	
≈ 3/4	Shoulder flexion/extension	≈ 3/4	
≈ 3/4	Shoulder abd/add	≈ 3/4	
WFL/≈ 3/4	Shoulder IR/ER	WFL/≈ 1/2	
≈ 3/4	Shoulder horizontal abd/add	≈ 1/2	
≈ 1/2/WFL	Elbow flexion/extension	≈ 1/2/WFL	
WFL	Forearm pronation/supination	WFL	

Table 2-12 continued

Left	Joint/Joint Complexes	Right	Comments
≈ 3/4	Wrist flexion/extension	≈ 3/4	
≈ 3/4	MCP flexion/extension	≈ 3/4	
≈ 3/4	PIP flexion/extension	≈ 3/4	
≈ 3/4	DIP flexion/extension	≈ 3/4	
≈ 3/4	Finger abd/add	≈ 3/4	
≈ 3/4	Thumb MCP flexion/extension	≈ 3/4	
≈ 3/4	Thumb ICP flexion/extension	≈ 3/4	
≈ 3/4	Thumb abd/add	≈ 3/4	
≈ 3/4	Thumb opposition	≈ 3/4	
	Lower Extremities		
≈ 3/4	SLR	≈ 3/4	
≈ 3/4/WFL	Hip flexion/extension	≈ 3/4/ WFL	
≈ 1/2/WFL	Hip abd/add	≈ 1/2/ WFL	
WFL/ ≈ 1/2	Hip IR/ER	WFL/≈ 1/2	
≈ 3/4/WFL	Knee flexion/extension	≈ 3/4/WFL	
≈ 1/2	Ankle plantar/dorsiflexion	≈ 1/2	
≈ 1/4	Foot eversion/inversion	≈ 1/4	
≈ 1/4	Great toe flexion/extension	≈ 1/4	
≈ 1/4	Toe MTP flexion/extension	≈ 1/4	
≈ 1/4	Toe IP flexion/extension	≈ 1/4	

abd = abduction; add = adduction; IR = internal rotation; ER = external rotation; MCP = metacarpophalangeal; PIP = proximal interphalangeal; DIP = distal interphalangeal; ICP = intermittent compression pump; WFL = within functional limits; ≈ = approximately.

Table 2-13

Manual Muscle Test

Left	Muscle/Muscle Group	Right	Comments
	Neck		
P+	Flexion/extension	P+	
P	Rotation	P	
P+	Lateral flexion	P+	

Table 2-13 continued

Left	Muscle/Muscle Group	Right	Comments
	Trunk		
P+	Flexion/extension	P+	
P	Rotation	P	
P+	Lateral flexion	P+	
P+	Pelvic elevation	P+	
	Upper Extremities		
P+	Scapular abd/add	P+	
P+	Scapular elevation	P+	
P+	Shoulder flexion/extension	P+	
P+	Shoulder abd/add	P+	
P+	Shoulder IR/ER	P+	
P+	Shoulder horizontal abd/add	P+	
F	Elbow flexion/extension	F	
F	Forearm pronation/supination	F	
F/P+	Wrist flexion/extension	F/P+	
F/P+	MCP flexion/extension	F/P+	
F/P+	PIP flexion/extension	F/P+	
F/P+	DIP flexion/extension	F/P+	
F/P+	Finger abd/add	F/P+	
F/P+	Thumb MCP flexion/extension	F/P+	
F/P+	Thumb ICP flexion/extension	F/P+	
F/P+	Thumb abd/add	F/P+	
F/P+	Thumb opposition	F/P+	
	Lower Extremities		
P+/F	Hip flexion/extension	P+/F	
P+/F	Hip abd/add	P+/F	
F/P+	Hip IR/ER	F/P+	
P+/F	Knee flexion/extension	P+/F	
P+	Ankle plantar/dorsiflexion	P+	
P+	Foot eversion/inversion	P+	
P+	Great toe flexion/extension	P+	

Table 2-13 continued			
Left	**Muscle/Muscle Group**	**Right**	**Comments**
P+	Toe MTP flexion/extension	P+	
P+	Toe IP flexion/extension	P+	

abd = abduction; add = adduction; IR = internal rotation; ER = external rotation; MCP = metacarpophalangeal; PIP = proximal interphalangeal; DIP = distal interphalangeal; ICP = intermittent compression pump; WNL = within normal limits; WFL = within functional limits; SLR = straight leg raise; G = good (80%); G+ = good (90%); F = fair (50%); F+ = fair (60%); F- = fair (40%); P = poor (20%); P+ = poor (30%); P- = poor (10%).

6. If both occupational and physical therapy were involved with this patient, what would you see as the role for each discipline to provide an appropriate, comprehensive treatment program? Consider the concepts of cotreatment and expert consultation in your answer.

7. Based upon the pathology that the patient exhibits and the individual impairments and functional limitations, do you think the patient will ever become totally "able" again? If not, which disabilities may remain?

8. What compensatory strategies might you teach the patient in this case?

9. What type(s) of DME (orthotic, prosthetic, or adaptive equipment) might you prescribe and why?

10. What would you propose as an appropriate treatment frequency and length of stay for this patient in your treatment setting? Provide the rationale for your answer.

11. What modifications would you have to make to the plan of care if you received insurance approval for only one-half of the time requested and the patient did not want to fund therapy privately?

12. Which portion(s) of the plan of care would you delegate to an assistant? Which portion(s) to an aide/tech? Provide your rationale for your answer.

13. For physical therapy students: Using the *Guidelines for Practice*, what would be your physical therapy diagnosis for this patient?

14. What environment(s) would you choose for implementing your treatment activities?

15. What activities would you use to address this patient's values?

16. Who is this patient? What roles and activities are important to him?

17. Give at least three strategies you could use to assist this patient and his family in dealing with his terminal illness and allow him to die with dignity.

EXERCISES FOR THE ASSISTANT STUDENT

Case #9: Martin VanWilkinson

1. Using the Nagi scheme of disability, present the active pathology (ies), impairments, functional limitations, and disabilities for this case.

2. Design a treatment session lasting 30 minutes for this patient.

3. If both occupational and physical therapy were involved with this patient, what would you see as the role for each discipline to provide an appropriate, comprehensive treatment program? Consider the concepts of cotreatment and expert consultation in your answer.

4. Based upon the pathology that the patient exhibits and the individual impairments and functional limitations, do you think the patient will ever become totally "able" again? If not, which disabilities may remain?

5. What compensatory strategies might you teach the patient in this case?

6. What type(s) of DME (orthotic, prosthetic, or adaptive equipment) might you prescribe and why?

7. Which portion(s) of the plan of care would you delegate to an aide/tech? Provide your rationale for your answer.

8. What environment(s) would you choose for implementing your treatment activities?

9. What activities would you use to address this patient's values?

10. Who is this patient? What roles and activities are important to him?

11. Give at least three strategies you could use to assist this patient and his family in dealing with his terminal illness and allow him to die with dignity.

Right Cerebrovascular Accident

At the age of 58, Marc Holliston was quite pleased with how his life was going. He was one of the top 10 brokers in his firm. He was filled with great pride when younger brokers referred to him to measure their success. All was well on the home front as well. His wife of 35 years, Margie, had always stood by him and managed their home and community obligations. Things were not always this smooth. Their 25-year-old son had a rough time "finding himself" after high school and ran into some trouble with the law. Now he is working and going to college at night. Marc was glad his son lived with them. It allowed him and his wife to keep a close eye on him. Also, his son was a big help. Margie's mother had moved in with them about a year ago because of her dementia. She is quite physically independent but requires supervision.

Over the years, Marc developed several medical problems. He has angina, atrial fibrillation (A-fib), HTN, and insulin-dependent diabetes mellitus (IDDM). Three years ago he had a hernia repair and he has not been able to quit smoking cigarettes (one to two packs a day since he was 16). He takes NPH insulin, Catapres, and nitroglycerin tabs prn.

Although he loves his work, he also enjoys his leisure time. He can be found in his box seats for all the baseball games whooping it up with the crowd. He also enjoys spending time with his wife on their powerboat during the summer season. At night, he can be found reading the evening newspaper and listening to the news at the same time. He enjoys his contemporary ranch-style home. It has four bedrooms and three bathrooms. The master suite has its own bathroom with a tub and shower stall. The home has no architectural barriers once inside. The home can be entered by four steps without a rail in the front or by the back, which has six railed steps.

One early afternoon while at work, Marc found himself feeling dizzy and nauseated. He tried to rest but the feeling did not go away. All he can recall is all of a sudden not being able to feel anything in his left arm and leg. He reports falling over because of his lack of control over his body. The next thing he remembers is waking up in the hospital. His wife was there along with his doctor, who was telling them that he had had a stroke. The CVA involved his right middle cerebral artery.

At this point, he complained about feeling exhausted and his need to get back on his feet to return to work. He had so much to accomplish.

After 10 days in acute care, Mr. Holliston was transferred to your transitional care unit with orders for evaluation and treatment to regain maximal functional abilities. His wife and son want Marc to return home. They would like him to achieve at least moderate assisted transfers so he can be assisted by them and whomever they may hire. Marc does not really appreciate many of his problems and hopes to return to work after a month of rehabilitation.

The results of the initial evaluation are as follows:

1. *Perception/cognition*: Severe left neglect complicated by hemisensory loss.

Cognition:
- *Alert and oriented x 3 using environmental cues (ie, room clock, calendar). Gives global reason for why he is hospitalized but is unaware of the severity.*
- *Attention: Demonstrates vigilance but easily distracted by the presence of others, especially family.*
- *Concentration: Inconsistent sustained concentration. Initially good but easily fatigues, as seen with increasing errors in performance; little recognition of errors.*
- *Memory: Long-term memory appears intact. Impaired short-term memory and immediate recall.*
- *Sequencing: Impaired; more pronounced when task involves crossing midline or bilaterality.*
- *Ability to follow directions: Impaired as evident by difficulty with immediate recall. Does better with pictorial instructions.*
- *Initiation: Impulsive.*
- *Insight/judgment: Poor; speaks of returning to home and work within 1 month as if nothing has happened. Poor appreciation for his current deficits.*
- *Problem solving: Poor. Has difficulty recognizing problems.*

2. *Neurology*: There is no active return of either his LUE or LLE. Tone is severely impaired with hypotonicity throughout the left extremities and trunk. Sustained clonus is noted at the left ankle.

3. *Sensation/pain*: Sensation is severely impaired with zero out of 10 correct responses during testing of proprioception, light touch, pain, deep pressure, and hot/cold. Mr. Holliston has no complaints of pain.

4. *Skin/edema*: Stage II pressure sore is noted on the left greater trochanter. Otherwise, skin is intact with moderate left hand and ankle/foot edema.

5. *Balance*: Balance is poor with the need for maximum assistance x 2 to maintain upright sitting on the edge of the mat. Standing balance is not appropriate to test.

6. *Mobility:*

Bed mobility:
- *Rolling: Maximum assistance with maximum verbal cues.*
- *Bridging: Maximum assistance with maximum verbal cues.*
- *Supine ↔ sit: Maximum assistance with maximum verbal cues.*
- *Equipment: Trapeze, rails.*

Transfers:
- *Sit → stand: Maximum assistance x 2 with maximum verbal cues.*
- *Bed ↔ wheelchair: Maximum assistance x 2 with maximum verbal cues.*
- *Chair: Maximum assistance x 2 with maximum verbal cues.*

- *Toilet (commode)* ↔ *wheelchair: Maximum assistance x 2 with maximum verbal cues.*
- *Tub/shower* ↔ *wheelchair: Maximum assistance x 2 with maximum verbal cues.*
- *Car: NT*

7. *Wheelchair mobility*: He requires total assistance for wheelchair propulsion and maneuvering due to impulsive behavior and left neglect. He requires wheelchair modifications to maintain his upright positioning in his wheelchair.

8. *Gait/functional mobility*: He is nonambulatory.

9. *Self-Care (right dominant):*

Feeding/equipment:

- *Requires complete set-up including cutting. Self feeds with pocketing, poor lip closure, and with great speed.*
- *Bathing: Maximum assistance dependent. Able to wash face after set-up; completes some grooming tasks and upper body washing, but not thoroughly. Left neglect evident.*
- *Grooming: Will try to comb hair, use electric razor, and brush teeth but impulsive and not thorough.*
- *Dressing: Maximum assistance with maximum cues for upper body. Impulsive, unable to carry over hemidressing techniques. Supported sitting. Dependent for his lower body, bed level.*
- *Toileting: Uses a urinal and bed pan. Maximum assistance required.*
- *Home management: NT.*
- *Leisure/community: Able to use portable programmed phone. He calls his contacts and friends to assure them he plans to return to work.*

10. *ROM*: See Table 2-14.

11. *Strength*: See Table 2-15.

PATIENT GOALS

1. Return to prior level of functioning.

FAMILY GOALS

1. Self feeding with minimal assistance.
2. Functional transfers with moderate assistance. Family to hire a personal care attendant.
3. Moderate assistance with toileting.
4. Moderate assistance with self-care.
5. Edema control.

EXERCISES FOR THE OT AND PT STUDENT

Case #10: Marc Holliston

1. Using the Nagi scheme of disability, present the active pathology(ies), impairments, functional limitations, and disabilities for this case.

2. Do you think the patient's goals are realistic? Why or why not? If not, what strategies would you use to help the patient focus on more realistic goals?

3. Write an assessment and plan for the patient case(s) assigned. Include appropriate short-term and long-term goals.

4. Present a thorough plan of care for the case (ie, what specifically would you do with this patient and why?)

5. Design a treatment session lasting 30 minutes for this patient.

6. If both occupational and physical therapy were involved with this patient, what would you see as the role for each discipline to provide an appropriate, comprehensive treatment program? Consider the concepts of cotreatment and expert consultation in your answer.

7. Based upon the pathology that the patient exhibits and the individual impairments and functional limitations, do you think the patient will ever become totally "able" again? If not, which disabilities may remain?

8. What compensatory strategies might you teach the patient in this case?

9. What type(s) of DME (orthotic, prosthetic, or adaptive equipment) might you prescribe and why?

10. What would you propose as an appropriate treatment frequency and length of stay for this patient in your treatment setting? Provide the rationale for your answer.

11. What modifications would you have to make to the plan of care if you received insurance approval for only one-half of the time requested and the patient did not want to fund therapy privately?

12. Which portion(s) of the plan of care would you delegate to an assistant? Which portion(s) to an aide/tech? Provide your rationale for your answer.

13. For physical therapy students: Using the *Guidelines for Practice*, what would be your physical therapy diagnosis for this patient?

14. What environment(s) would you choose for implementing your treatment activities?

15. What activities would you use to address this patient's values?

Table 2-14

Range of Motion

Left	Joint/Joint Complexes	Right	Comments
	Neck		
WNL	Flexion/extension	WNL	
WNL	Rotation	WNL	
WNL	Lateral flexion	WNL	
	Trunk		
WNL	Flexion/extension	WNL	
WNL	Rotation	WNL	
WNL	Lateral flexion	WNL	
WNL	Pelvic elevation	WNL	
	Upper Extremities		
WFL	Scapular abd/add	WNL	
WNL	Scapular elevation	WNL	
WNL	Shoulder flexion/extension	WNL	
WNL	Shoulder abd/add	WNL	
WNL	Shoulder IR/ER	WNL	
WNL	Shoulder horizontal abd/add	WNL	
WNL	Elbow flexion/extension	WNL	
WNL	Forearm pronation/supination	WNL	
WNL	Wrist flexion/extension	WNL	
WNL	MCP flexion/extension	WNL	
WNL	PIP flexion/extension	WNL	
WNL	DIP flexion/extension	WNL	
WNL	Finger abd/add	WNL	
WNL	Thumb MCP flexion/extension	WNL	
WNL	Thumb ICP flexion/extension	WNL	
WNL	Thumb abd/add	WNL	
WNL	Thumb opposition	WNL	
	Lower Extremities		
WNL	SLR	WNL	
WNL	Hip flexion/extension	WNL	
WNL	Hip abd/add	WNL	

Table 2-14 continued

Left	Joint/Joint Complexes	Right	Comments
WNL	Hip IR/ER	WNL	
WNL	Knee flexion/extension	WNL	
WNL	Ankle plantar/dorsiflexion	WNL	
WNL	Foot eversion/inversion	WNL	
WNL	Great toe flexion/extension	WNL	
WNL	Toe MTP flexion/extension	WNL	
WNL	Toe IP flexion/extension	WNL	

abd = abduction; add = adduction; IR = internal rotation; ER = external rotation; MCP = metacarpophalangeal; PIP = proximal interphalangeal; DIP = distal interphalangeal; ICP = intermittent compression pump; WNL = within normal limits; WFL = within functional limits.

Table 2-15

Manual Muscle Test

Left	Muscle/Muscle Group	Right	Comments
	Neck		
G	Flexion/extension	G-/G	
G	Rotation	G-/G	
G	Lateral flexion	G-/G	
	Trunk		
P+/F+	Flexion/extension	P+/F+	
P+/F+	Rotation	P+/F+	
P+/F+	Lateral flexion	P+/F+	
P+/F+	Pelvic elevation	P+/F+	
	Upper Extremities		
Trace	Scapular abd/add	G/N	
Trace	Scapular elevation	G/N	
0	Shoulder flexion/extension	G/N	
0	Shoulder abd/add	G/N	
0	Shoulder IR/ER	G/N	
0	Shoulder horizontal abd/add	G/N	
0	Elbow flexion/extension	G/N	
0	Forearm pronation/supination	G/N	

Table 2-15 continued

Left	Muscle/Muscle Group	Right	Comments
0	Wrist flexion/extension	G/N	
0	MCP flexion/extension	G/N	
0	PIP flexion/extension	G/N	
0	DIP flexion/extension	G/N	
0	Finger abd/add	G/N	
0	Thumb MCP flexion/extension	G/N	
0	Thumb ICP flexion/extension	G/N	
0	Thumb abd/add	G/N	
0	Thumb opposition	G/N	
	Lower Extremities		
0	Hip flexion/extension	G/N	
0	Hip abd/add	G/N	
0	Hip IR/ER	G/N	
0	Knee flexion/extension	G/N	
0	Ankle plantar/dorsiflexion	G/N	
0	Foot eversion/inversion	G/N	
0	Great toe flexion/extension	G/N	
0	Toe MTP flexion/extension	G/N	
0	Toe IP flexion/extension	G/N	

abd = abduction; add = adduction; IR = internal rotation; ER = external rotation; MCP = metacarpophalangeal; PIP = proximal interphalangeal; DIP = distal interphalangeal; ICP = intermittent compression pump; WNL = within normal limits; WFL = within functional limits; SLR = straight leg raise; G = good (80%); G+ = good (90%); F = fair (50%); F+ = fair (60%); F- = fair (40%); P = poor (20%); P+ = poor (30%); P- = poor (10%).

16. Who is this patient? What roles and activities are important to him?

17. What do you see as the role of the mental health practitioner in this case?

EXERCISES FOR THE ASSISTANT STUDENT

Case #10: Marc Holliston

1. Using the Nagi scheme of disability, present the active pathology(ies), impairments, functional limitations, and disabilities for this case.

2. Design a treatment session lasting 30 minutes for this patient.

3. If both occupational and physical therapy were involved with this patient, what would you see as the role for each discipline to provide an appropriate, comprehensive treatment program? Consider the concepts of cotreatment and expert consultation in your answer.

4. Based upon the pathology that the patient exhibits and the individual impairments and functional limitations, do you think the patient will ever become totally "able" again? If not, which disabilities may remain?

5. What compensatory strategies might you teach the patient in this case?

6. What type(s) of DME (orthotic, prosthetic, or adaptive equipment) might you prescribe and why?

7. Which portion(s) of the plan of care would you delegate to an aide/tech? Provide your rationale for your answer.

8. What environment(s) would you choose for implementing your treatment activities?

9. What activities would you use to address this patient's values?

10. Who is this patient? What roles and activities are important to him?

11. What do you see as the role of the mental health practitioner in this case?

Post-Polio Syndrome

Marvin Hewitt is a 64-year-old man who was diagnosed with polio at age 8 and with post-polio syndrome last year. He lives at home with his wife, who is 58 and his 24-year-old daughter. His 27-year-old son lives two blocks away with his wife and their two children, ages 3 and 5. Marvin believes that his life is nearly perfect, as his family is not only close geographically but close emotionally. His pride and joy are his grandchildren with whom he typically visits four to five times each week. He is currently a high school history teacher but plans to retire next year. He plans to spend his time volunteering for the ministries of his church as an English as a second language tutor, and as a fundraiser. As his wife does not work, she plans to join him in his endeavors. Currently, his leisure time is spent going to the movies, visiting museums, and dining out. He is very social and enjoys being with family and friends.

Prior to the onset of post-polio syndrome, he was independent in all activities of daily living and all aspects of mobility. He was the primary caretaker of the house and yard, often doing the major repairs. His wife took care of all indoor housekeeping responsibilities and did all of the cooking. Despite the setbacks from his post-polio syndrome he was able to maintain much of his independence, but due to rapid onset of muscle fatigue and weakness, especially in the lower extremities, he has had to hire help for major repairs and the heavier yardwork. He was able to continue to mow the lawn with a rider mower and maintain the small flower beds that line the walkway to his home.

Two weeks ago, he became ill with what he initially thought was a cold. His symptoms spread to his chest, and 4 days ago he was admitted to the hospital with pneumonia. He received intravenous antibiotics and respiratory therapy during this time and on the day of discharge was seen by physical and occupational therapy for brief evaluations. These clinicians, however, did not have time to gather more than the basic data to complete his referral to your skilled nursing facility.

He is now referred to your facility for subacute rehab after his hospitalization, as it is clear that he has had a tremendous decline in function and therefore cannot return home. This hospitalization and his worsening post-polio syndrome have left him functionally dependent. He was brought to your facility with orders for rehabilitation services to regain maximum mobility.

He presents to you with the following:

1. *Significant past medical history*: Polio at age 8 with minimal residual weakness requiring use of an AFO on his LLE and a cane for ambulation. HTN, pneumonia 2 years ago, cataract in the left eye, and s/p hernia repair 20 years ago.

2. *Medications*: Tylenol prn for complaints of muscle stiffness and pain, especially lower extremity distal muscles, and Tenormin. He takes a multivitamin daily.

3. *Cognition/perception*: He is alert and oriented x 3 with intact memory and intellect apparent. He does not demonstrate any perceptual deficits on gross examination.

4. *Sensation*: His sensation is intact for all modalities in all areas.

5. *ROM*: ROM is WNL for all extremities, neck, and trunk passively with the exception of a bilateral plantarflexion contracture of -5 degrees of dorsiflexion on the left and -10 degrees of dorsiflexion on the right.

6. *Strength*: See Table 2-16.

7. *Balance*: His sitting balance is normal. His standing balance is moderately impaired, requiring a walker and minimum assistance to attain and maintain upright. He does not tolerate more than minimal challenges to his balance in standing with a walker.

8. *Pain*: Patient has moderate, frequent complaints of lower extremity muscle stiffness and cramping. Otherwise without complaints of pain.

9. *Skin/edema*: Intact skin integrity. Moderate bilateral distal lower extremity edema with TED stockings worn.

10. *Mobility*:

Bed mobility:

- *Rolling: Independent side to side and supine to prone with significant effort.*
- *Bridging: Minimum assistance to complete a full bridge.*
- *Supine ↔ sit: Minimum assistance.*
- *Equipment: None at present.*

Transfers:

- *Sit → stand: Minimum assistance with rolling walker.*
- *Bed ↔ w/c: Minimum assistance with rolling walker.*
- *w/c ↔ commode: Minimum assistance with rolling walker.*
- *Toilet ↔ w/c: Moderate assistance with a three-in-one commode over the toilet secondary to limited space for assistive device.*
- *Tub/shower: NT.*
- *Car: NT.*

11. *Gait:* He is able to ambulate 100 feet with a rolling walker with minimum assistance using his left AFO (although fit is marginal due to new plantarflexor contractures), however, frequent posterior loss of balance is noted with occasional knee buckling on the right.

Table 2-16

Manual Muscle Test

Left	Muscle/Muscle Group	Right	Comments
	Neck		
G-	Flexion/extension	G-	
G-	Rotation	G-	
G-	Lateral flexion	G-	
	Trunk		
P+	Flexion/extension	P+	Tested functionally
F-	Rotation	F-	
F-	Lateral flexion	F-	
F-	Pelvic elevation	F-	
	Upper Extremities		
WFL	Scapular abd/add	WFL	
WFL	Scapular elevation	WFL	
WFL	Shoulder flexion/extension	WFL	
WFL	Shoulder abd/add	WFL	
WFL	Shoulder IR/ER	WFL	
WFL	Shoulder horizontal abd/add	WFL	
WFL	Elbow flexion/extension	WFL	
WFL	Forearm pronation/supination	WFL	
WFL	Wrist flexion/extension	WFL	
WFL	MCP flexion/extension	WFL	
WFL	PIP flexion/extension	WFL	
WFL	DIP flexion/extension	WFL	
WFL	Finger abd/add	WFL	
WFL	Thumb MCP flexion/extension	WFL	
WFL	Thumb ICP flexion/extension	WFL	
WFL	Thumb abd/add	WFL	
WFL	Thumb opposition	WFL	
	Lower Extremities		
F/P+	Hip flexion/extension	F-/P+	
P+	Hip abd/add	P+	
F	Hip IR/ER	F	

Table 2-16 continued

Left	Muscle/Muscle Group	Right	Comments
F/F	Knee flexion/extension	F/F-	
P+/F-	Ankle plantar/dorsiflexion	P+/P+	
F-/F-	Foot eversion/inversion	F-/F-	
F-/F-	Great toe flexion/extension	F-/P	
F-/F-	Toe MTP flexion/extension	F-/F-	
F-/F-	Toe IP flexion/extension	F-/F-	

abd = abduction; add = adduction; IR = internal rotation; ER = external rotation; MCP = metacarpophalangeal; PIP = proximal interphalangeal; DIP = distal interphalangeal; ICP = intermittent compression pump; WNL = within normal limits; WFL = within functional limits; SLR = straight leg raise; G = good (80%); G+ = good (90%); F = fair (50%); F+ = fair (60%); F- = fair (40%); P = poor (20%); P+ = poor (30%); P- = poor (10%).

12. *Functional mobility*: This patient is independent in wheel-chair set-up, propulsion, and maneuvering on level, indoor surfaces to complete basic functional tasks. He requires minimum to moderate assistance when ambulating with a rolling walker and fatigues quickly, making this mode of mobility dysfunctional at present.

13. *Self-care*: He is independent in most aspects of self-care from a seated position including feeding, grooming, and upper body dressing. He is able to complete most lower body dressing but requires moderate assistance for stand-hike to don underwear and pants. He requires moderate assistance for toileting.

14. *Home management*: This individual is dependent for the home management tasks that he was responsible for prior to the onset of his illness.

PATIENT GOALS

1. Independent transfers with AFO and straight cane.
2. Independent lower body dressing.
3. Independent toileting.
4. Independent showering.
3. Independent ambulation with AFO and straight cane sufficient to return to home and work activities.
4. Return to work.
5. Return to driving.

EXERCISES FOR THE OT AND PT STUDENT

Case #11: Marvin Hewitt

1. Using the Nagi scheme of disability, present the active pathology(ies), impairments, functional limitations, and disabilities for this case.

2. Do you think the patient's goals are realistic? Why or why not? If not, what strategies would you use to help the patient focus on more realistic goals?

3. Write an assessment and plan for the patient case(s) assigned. Include appropriate short-term and long-term goals.

4. Present a thorough plan of care for the case (ie, what specifically would you do with this patient and why?)

5. Design a treatment session lasting 30 minutes for this patient.

6. If both occupational and physical therapy were involved with this patient, what would you see as the role for each discipline to provide an appropriate, comprehensive treatment program? Consider the concepts of cotreatment and expert consultation in your answer.

7. Based upon the pathology that the patient exhibits and the individual impairments and functional limitations, do you think the patient will ever become totally "able" again? If not, which disabilities may remain?

8. What compensatory strategies might you teach the patient in this case?

9. What type(s) of DME (orthotic, prosthetic, or adaptive equipment) might you prescribe and why?

10. What would you propose as an appropriate treatment frequency and length of stay for this patient in your treatment setting? Provide the rationale for your answer.

11. What modifications would you have to make to the plan of care if you received insurance approval for only one-half of the time requested and the patient did not want to fund therapy privately?

12. Which portion(s) of the plan of care would you delegate to an assistant? Which portion(s) to an aide/tech? Provide your rationale for your answer.

13. For physical therapy students: Using the *Guidelines for Practice*, what would be your physical therapy diagnosis for this patient?

14. What environment(s) would you choose for implementing your treatment activities?

15. What activities would you use to address this patient's values?

16. Who is this patient? What roles and activities are important to him?

17. What are the current research findings regarding exercise for the individual with post-polio syndrome?

EXERCISES FOR THE ASSISTANT STUDENT

Case #11: Marvin Hewitt

1. Using the Nagi scheme of disability, present the active pathology(ies), impairments, functional limitations, and disabilities for this case.

2. Design a treatment session lasting 30 minutes for this patient.

3. If both occupational and physical therapy were involved with this patient, what would you see as the role for each discipline to provide an appropriate, comprehensive treatment program? Consider the concepts of cotreatment and expert consultation in your answer.

4. Based upon the pathology that the patient exhibits and the individual impairments and functional limitations, do you think the patient will ever become totally "able" again? If not, which disabilities may remain?

5. What compensatory strategies might you teach the patient in this case?

6. What type(s) of DME (orthotic, prosthetic, or adaptive equipment) might you prescribe and why?

7. Which portion(s) of the plan of care would you delegate to an aide/tech? Provide your rationale for your answer.

8. What environment(s) would you choose for implementing your treatment activities?

9. What activities would you use to address this patient's values?

10. Who is this patient? What roles and activities are important to him?

11. What are the current research findings regarding exercise for the individual with post-polio syndrome?

Spinal Cord Injury

Kathy Robinson is a 43-year-old divorced mother of two children. She has an 8-year-old son and a 6-year-old daughter. Daily, she juggles her life to meet all of its demands. She works full-time as the chief financial officer of a midsized software company. Also, she is the primary parent for her children. She has hired part-time household help to pick up her children and assist with some of the household management. Kathy relieves her stress by participating in cardio fitness classes three to five times each week.

Kathy and her children live in a three-bedroom condo, which is all on one level. The unit has one and one-half standard bathrooms. The kitchen has a standard "L" shape design. There are four steps without rails leading to the front door to enter the home. The back door has six steps with a rail.

While Kathy was a passenger in her friend's car, a vehicle that ran a red light struck them. Kathy was diagnosed with a T-11 spinal fracture, which resulted in a complete spinal cord injury (SCI). She was discharged to your rehabilitation center 5 weeks later after having surgery for Harrington rod placement. She has orders for evaluation and treatment to regain maximum activities of daily living (ADL), mobility, and transfer status. Currently, she is receiving baclofen to manage her tone and darvon for pain.

Upon admission she expresses her feelings of despair and of being overwhelmed by her situation. She fears not being able to return to her prior life roles, especially as the primary caregiver for her children.

The results of Ms. Robinson's initial evaluation are as follows:

1. *Perception*: WNL. The patient wears contacts for nearsightedness.

2. *Cognition*: WNL.

3. *Neurology*: Moderate to severe spasticity of bilateral lower extremity (BLE) has been an issue. Baclofen has been prescribed by her physician.

4. *Sensation/pain*: Sensation is absent below the level of the lesion. Otherwise it is completely intact. She does have some complaints of palmar sensitivity due to wheelchair mobility. She also has frequent complaints of moderate pain throughout her upper back.

5. *Skin/edema*: Unremarkable; TED worn secondary to immobility.

6. *Balance*: Balance is poor in sitting, with patient able to sit when assisted to attain sitting position with a BUE supporting her on the mat or with a bedside table in front of her.

7. *Mobility:*

Bed mobility:

- *Rolling: Moderate assistance with half-rails.*
- *Bridging: Unable.*
- *Supine ↔ sit: Moderate assistance.*
- *Equipment: Rails.*

Transfers:

- *Sit → stand: NT.*
- *Bed ↔ wheelchair: Maximum assistance with slide board.*
- *Chair: N/A.*
- *Toilet ↔ wheelchair: Maximum assistance with slide board commode.*
- *Tub/shower ↔ wheelchair: Maximum assistance with transfer bench.*
- *Car: NT.*

8. *Wheelchair mobility*: She is independent with short-distance wheelchair mobility (1000 feet) on level, open areas. Also, she is independent with maneuvering but this is slow and deliberate and not functional at this time. She requires minimal assistance on ramps; curbs have not yet been assessed.

9. *Self-care:*

- *Feeding/equipment: Independent.*
- *Bathing: Independent with all upper body tasks. She bathes her lower body, bed level, using adaptive equipment (leg lifter and long-handled sponge). She requires moderate assistance for lower body tasks.*
- *Grooming: Independent.*
- *Dressing: Independent with all upper body tasks. Dresses her lower body, bed level, using adaptive equipment (leg lifter) with moderate assistance. She requires maximal assistance for footwear.*
- *Toileting: Bowel and bladder programs need to be addressed. She requires maximal assistance for all toileting activities.*
- *Home management: To be assessed at wheelchair level.*
- *Leisure/community: Patient states that she does not have the ability to be involved in any activities at this time.*

10. *ROM*: See Table 2-17.

11. *Strength*: See Table 2-18.

PATIENT GOALS

1. Independent self-care, including toileting.
2. Independent bed mobility.
3. Independent transfers to all surfaces.
4. Independent wheelchair mobility at home and in the community.
5. Return to caring for her children.
6. Independent household management.
7. Return to driving.
8. Return to work.

EXERCISES FOR THE OT AND PT STUDENT

Case #13: Kathy Robinson

1. Using the Nagi scheme of disability, present the active pathology(ies), impairments, functional limitations, and disabilities for this case.

2. Do you think the patient's goals are realistic? Why or why not? If not, what strategies would you use to help the patient focus on more realistic goals?

3. Write an assessment and plan for the patient case(s) assigned. Include appropriate short-term and long-term goals.

4. Present a thorough plan of care for the case (ie, what specifically would you do with this patient and why?)

5. Design a treatment session lasting 30 minutes for this patient.

6. If both occupational and physical therapy were involved with this patient, what would you see as the role for each discipline to provide an appropriate, comprehensive treatment program? Consider the concepts of cotreatment and expert consultation in your answer.

7. Based upon the pathology that the patient exhibits and the individual impairments and functional limitations, do you think the patient will ever become totally "able" again? If not, which disabilities may remain?

8. What compensatory strategies might you teach the patient in this case?

9. What type(s) of DME (orthotic, prosthetic, or adaptive equipment) might you prescribe and why?

10. What would you propose as an appropriate treatment frequency and length of stay for this patient in your treatment setting? Provide the rationale for your answer.

11. What modifications would you have to make to the plan of care if you received insurance approval for only one-half of the time requested and the patient did not want to fund therapy privately?

12. Which portion(s) of the plan of care would you delegate to an assistant? Which portion(s) to an aide/tech? Provide your rationale for your answer.

13. For physical therapy students: Using the *Guidelines for Practice*, what would be your physical therapy diagnosis for this patient?

14. What environment(s) would you choose for implementing your treatment activities?

15. What activities would you use to address this patient's values?

<u>Table 2-17</u>

Range of Motion

Left	Joint/Joint Complexes	Right	Comments
	Neck		
WNL	Flexion/extension	WNL	
WNL	Rotation	WNL	
WNL	Lateral flexion	WNL	
	Trunk		
NT	Flexion/extension	NT	Patient is immobilized in a body jacket
	Rotation		
	Lateral flexion		
	Pelvic elevation		
	Upper Extremities		
WNL	Scapular abd/add	WNL	
WNL	Scapular elevation		
WNL	Shoulder flexion/extension	WNL	
WNL	Shoulder abd/add	WNL	
WNL	Shoulder IR/ER	WNL	
WNL	Shoulder horizontal abd/add	WNL	
WNL	Elbow flexion/extension	WNL	
WNL	Forearm pronation/supination	WNL	
WNL	Wrist flexion/extension	WNL	
WNL	MCP flexion/extension	WNL	
WNL	PIP flexion/extension	WNL	
WNL	DIP flexion/extension	WNL	
WNL	Finger abd/add	WNL	
WNL	Thumb MCP flexion/extension	WNL	
WNL	Thumb ICP flexion/extension	WNL	
WNL	Thumb abd/add	WNL	
WNL	Thumb opposition	WNL	
	Lower Extremities		
WNL	SLR	WNL	
WNL	Hip flexion/extension	WNL	
WNL	Hip abd/add	WNL	

Table 2-17 continued

Left	Joint/Joint Complexes	Right	Comments
WNL	Hip IR/ER	WNL	
WNL	Knee flexion/extension	WNL	
WNL	Ankle plantar/dorsiflexion	WNL	
WNL	Foot eversion/inversion	WNL	
WNL	Great toe flexion/extension	WNL	
WNL	Toe MTP flexion/extension	WNL	
WNL	Toe IP flexion/extension	WNL	

abd = abduction; add = adduction; IR = internal rotation; ER = external rotation; MCP = metacarpophalangeal; PIP = proximal interphalangeal; DIP = distal interphalangeal; ICP = intermittent compression pump; WNL = within normal limits; WFL = within functional limits; NT = not tested.

Table 2-18

Manual Muscle Test

Left	Muscle/Muscle Group	Right	Comments
	Neck		
G/N	Flexion/extension	G/N	
G/N	Rotation	G/N	
G/N	Lateral flexion	G/N	
	Trunk		
NT	Flexion/extension	NT	
NT	Rotation	NT	
NT	Lateral flexion	NT	
NT	Pelvic elevation	NT	
	Upper Extremities		
G/N	Scapular abd/add	G/N	
G/N	Scapular elevation	G/N	
G/N	Shoulder flexion/extension	G/N	
G/N	Shoulder abd/add	G/N	
G/N	Shoulder IR/ER	G/N	
G/N	Shoulder horizontal abd/add	G/N	
G/N	Elbow flexion/extension	G/N	
G/N	Forearm pronation/supination	G/N	

Table 2-18 continued

Left	Muscle/Muscle Group	Right	Comments
G/N	Wrist flexion/extension	G/N	
G/N	MCP flexion/extension	G/N	
G/N	PIP flexion/extension	G/N	
G/N	DIP flexion/extension	G/N	
G/N	Finger abd/add	G/N	
G/N	Thumb MCP flexion/extension	G/N	
G/N	Thumb ICP flexion/extension	G/N	
G/N	Thumb abd/add	G/N	
G/N	Thumb opposition	G/N	
	Lower Extremities		
0	Hip flexion/extension	0	
0	Hip abd/add	0	
0	Hip IR/ER	0	
0	Knee flexion/extension	0	
0	Ankle plantar/dorsiflexion	0	
0	Foot eversion/inversion	0	
0	Great toe flexion/extension	0	
0	Toe MTP flexion/extension	0	
0	Toe IP flexion/extension	0	

abd = abduction; add = adduction; IR = internal rotation; ER = external rotation; MCP = metacarpophalangeal; PIP = proximal interphalangeal; DIP = distal interphalangeal; ICP = intermittent compression pump; WNL = within normal limits; WFL = within functional limits; SLR = straight leg raise; G = good (80%); G+ = good (90%); F = fair (50%); F+ = fair (60%); F- = fair (40%); P = poor (20%); P+ = poor (30%); P- = poor (10%).

16. Who is this patient? What roles and activities are important to her?

17. How might this individual be able to return to aerobic exercise to meet her leisure needs?

EXERCISES FOR THE ASSISTANT STUDENT

Case #13: Kathy Robinson

1. Using the Nagi scheme of disability, present the active pathology(ies), impairments, functional limitations, and disabilities for this case.

2. Design a treatment session lasting 30 minutes for this patient.

3. If both occupational and physical therapy were involved with this patient, what would you see as the role for each discipline to provide an appropriate, comprehensive treatment program? Consider the concepts of cotreatment and expert consultation in your answer.

4. Based upon the pathology that the patient exhibits and the individual impairments and functional limitations, do you think the patient will ever become totally "able" again? If not, which disabilities may remain?

5. What compensatory strategies might you teach the patient in this case?

6. What type(s) of DME (orthotic, prosthetic, or adaptive equipment) might you prescribe and why?

7. Which portion(s) of the plan of care would you delegate to an aide/tech? Provide your rationale for your answer.

8. What environment(s) would you choose for implementing your treatment activities?

9. What activities would you use to address this patient's values?

10. Who is this patient? What roles and activities are important to her?

11. How might this individual be able to return to aerobic exercise to meet her leisure needs?

Traumatic Brain Injury

Sarah Johnson is a healthy 57-year-old grandmother of three. She is an enthusiastic homemaker and enjoys bike riding and quilting. She is active in her church and makes baby clothes that are donated to the needy. Every year, Sarah plans and expands her annual flower beds. When her husband retires, they hope to winter in a warmer climate and have their adult children tend to their two story colonial they've lived in for many years.

Sarah's husband, Charlie, works full-time in maintenance for a high tech company. He tends to the lawn, garbage, and washes the supper dishes. If asked, they both feel content with their current lifestyle.

During a usual bike ride to visit her grandchildren, Sarah is struck by a car. When the medical response team arrives, she is able to move her extremities but appears confused and has no recall of the accident. Also, she is unable to give her personal information. It takes several hours before her identity is established.

At the local hospital, she is diagnosed with a traumatic brain injury with amnesia for the events prior and after her injury. Sarah moves and speaks haltingly. She complains of a constant severe headache and numerous body pains. Her skin has many abrasions and contusions with two black eyes.

Her family's response is to rally to her side and pledges to do whatever it takes to return Sarah to her prior level of health and functioning. Her spouse appears immobilized by the recent events and his children need to take charge of the situation and his care.

At a meeting with the hospital's social worker, Sarah's daughter requests that her mother receive rehabilitation for her cognitive changes. She states that her father needs her mother to be the person that she was and that because of personal circumstances with her own young family she did not have much time to help out.

Plans were made for Sarah to be transferred to an acute rehabilitation center.

These are the findings of her initial evaluation:

1. *Past medical history*: For the most part insignificant. She has a family history of diabetes and she was monitoring her dietary intake.

2. *Perception*: Appears WFL. However, patient exhibits perseveration while scanning and she requires minimum cues to locate objects. She also requires moderate cues to locate environmental cues for topographical orientation within the hospital.

3. *Cognition*: Oriented to self and is able to identify family members. Is unable to give detailed information about her family (ie, birthdates of her grandchildren). She initiates the use of environmental cues (ie, calendars or clocks) for time. She is able to attend to concrete tasks in a quiet, non-stimulating environment for about 10 minutes. She exhibits difficulty with divided attention and abstract tasks. This is evident when asked to gather toiletries and clothing for self-care. She wanders around looking for items randomly. She has difficulty articulating her plan. However, when asked structured questions (ie, what do you put on first and what do you need to do it?) she is able to perform. She also needs to be called back to a task if there is an interruption or if distracted by an item. Sarah has difficulty recalling what items are located behind closed doors and drawers. A basic memory book has been instituted for Sarah. It includes why she is at the rehabilitation center, a calendar, daily schedule, and notes from people that have interacted with her. She is able to problem solve in concrete situations when cued 50% of the time.

4. *ROM*: Limited by pain.

5. *Neurology*: Sensation, tone, strength, and balance are intact but are slow to react.

6. *Pain*: Experiences muscle pain from the accident, along with pain due to abrasions and contusions.

7. *Skin*: Multiple contusions and abrasions over head, trunk, and extremities.

8. *Mobility*: Ambulates without a device. Moves slowly. However, needs moderate cues to locate destination if not visible (ie, closed bathroom door).

9. *Transfers*: Uses versa frame for safety during toilet transfers and tub seat for showering. Requires moderate cues for carryover of tub transfer technique.

10. *Self-care*: Independent with eating.

   - *Bathing: Moderate cues to gather items. Requires moderate verbal cueing to complete if she is distracted.*

   - *Dressing: Moderate cueing to generate a plan to locate items. Able to self dress.*

   - *Toileting: Independent with toileting hygiene and clothing management.*

   - *Grooms: Minimum cues to sequence.*

11. *Home management*: Minimum cues to complete a brownie mix after set-up. Moderate cues for baking due to safety issues. Supervised for bed making.

PATIENT/FAMILY GOALS

1. To return home.

2. To be independent with self-care.

3. To be independent with toileting.

4. Not to need adaptive equipment.

5. To be left home alone during the day while husband works.

6. To be able to prepare light meals.

7. To be able to complete home management.

EXERCISES FOR THE OT AND PT STUDENT

Case #14: Sarah Johnson

1. Using the Nagi scheme of disability, present the active pathology(ies), impairments, functional limitations, and disabilities for this case.

2. Do you think the patient's goals are realistic? Why or why not? If not, what strategies would you use to help the patient focus on more realistic goals?

3. Write an assessment and plan for the patient case(s) assigned. Include appropriate short-term and long-term goals.

4. Present a thorough plan of care for the case (ie, what specifically would you do with this patient and why?)

5. Design a treatment session lasting 30 minutes for this patient.

6. If both occupational and physical therapy were involved with this patient, what would you see as the role for each discipline to provide an appropriate, comprehensive treatment program? Consider the concepts of cotreatment and expert consultation in your answer.

7. Based upon the pathology that the patient exhibits and the individual impairments and functional limitations, do you think the patient will ever become totally "able" again? If not, which disabilities may remain?

8. What compensatory strategies might you teach the patient in this case?

9. What type(s) of DME (orthotic, prosthetic, or adaptive equipment) might you prescribe and why?

10. What would you propose as an appropriate treatment frequency and length of stay for this patient in your treatment setting? Provide the rationale for your answer.

11. What modifications would you have to make to the plan of care if you received insurance approval for only one-half of the time requested and the patient did not want to fund therapy privately?

12. Which portion(s) of the plan of care would you delegate to an assistant? Which portion(s) to an aide/tech? Provide your rationale for your answer.

13. For physical therapy students: Using the *Guidelines for Practice*, what would be your physical therapy diagnosis for this patient?

14. What environment(s) would you choose for implementing your treatment activities?

15. What activities would you use to address this patient's values?

16. Who is this patient? What roles and activities are important to her?

17. What do you think Sarah's daughter's role should be during the rehabilitation process?

EXERCISES FOR THE ASSISTANT STUDENT

Case #14: Sarah Johnson

1. Using the Nagi scheme of disability, present the active pathology (ies), impairments, functional limitations, and disabilities for this case.

2. Design a treatment session lasting 30 minutes for this patient.

3. If both occupational and physical therapy were involved with this patient, what would you see as the role for each discipline to provide an appropriate, comprehensive treatment program? Consider the concepts of cotreatment and expert consultation in your answer.

4. Based upon the pathology that the patient exhibits and the individual impairments and functional limitations, do you think the patient will ever become totally "able" again? If not, which disabilities may remain?

5. What compensatory strategies might you teach the patient in this case?

6. What type(s) of DME (orthotic, prosthetic, or adaptive equipment) might you prescribe and why?

7. Which portion(s) of the plan of care would you delegate to an aide/tech? Provide your rationale for your answer.

8. What environment(s) would you choose for implementing your treatment activities?

9. What activities would you use to address this patient's values?

10. Who is this patient? What roles and activities are important to her?

11. What do you think Sarah's daughter's role should be during the rehabilitation process?

RHEUMATOLOGY 3

Osteoarthritis

By the age of 67, Edna Marcusso had learned to adapt to her changing health status. She has a long history of HTN, osteoarthritis, and osteoporosis. About 2 years ago, she had been diagnosed with emphysema and many of her daily activities became increasingly laborious. In spite of her breathing difficulties, she continued to smoke and proceeded with her routines, slowly. Her husband would pitch in to help her when she was feeling especially slow or short of breath.

A year later, she decided to retire from her long tenure as an executive secretary for a small manufacturing company. This allowed her the time and energy to pursue her interests—family and friends. At this time, she continued to be an active participant in household management. She was responsible for the cleaning, shopping, laundry, and meal preparation at home. Volunteering at the local hospital fulfilled her sense of contributing to her community. As time went on, she noticed that she moved even more slowly. She assumed this was related to "normal" aging. However, when she began to experience generalized pain in her right hip, she became alarmed.

At this point, Edna made an appointment with her physician. Her pain and difficulty rising from a chair became increasingly difficult. She dreaded showering. The bathroom steam negatively affected her breathing and now she struggled to enter/exit the tub. She had always looked forward to her weekly shopping trips with friends. Now, she self-medicated with aspirin to control her pain when she had to get in/out of the car. She avoided her favorite mall, as she suffered to walk its length.

Her physician recommended a total hip replacement (THR). This procedure would let her resume her lifestyle. In order for the surgery to occur, Edna had to quit smoking. After some false starts, she was successful. By the time she was ready for the surgery her physical condition had declined. She had intensified pain and had gained 20 pounds. She began using a wheelchair for community mobility and had placed many of her interests on hold.

The actual procedure was completed as planned. Edna completed a short 10-day course in acute rehab and was referred to the local outpatient clinic for further therapy intervention. She has THP and is PWB.

On intake, she clearly states her goals as wanting to be independent with her self-care, including showering. She admits allowing her husband to complete her lower body tasks, "because it's easier." She wants to be independent with all transfers and to ambulate, preferably without a cane. She hopes to resume household tasks and all community activities. She reports that she and her husband live in a ranch-style home with one step to enter. The bathroom is standard and there are no other architectural barriers once inside the house.

The results of the initial evaluation are as follows:

1. *Perception*: Mrs. Marcusso wears eyeglasses. Otherwise perception is WNL.

2. *Cognition*: WNL. She is able to state her THP.

3. *Motor control*: WFL.

4. *Sensation/pain*: Intact sensation without any signs of neurologic deficit. Mrs. Marcusso states that prior arthritic pain was a 6 on a 1 to 10 scale at rest, and now she is pain free at rest. Pain with PROM/AROM of right hip is a 3 on a 1 to 10 scale.

5. *Skin/edema*: Clean, dry suture.

6. *Balance*: Intact static balance, sitting, and standing. Impaired dynamic sitting and standing balance secondary to parameters of THP. Uses long-handled LE equipment to extend reach.

7. *Mobility:*
   - *Bed mobility: Independent with good adherence to THP; uses adductor wedge.*

Transfers:
   - *Sit → stand: Independent with rolling walker.*
   - *Bed: Independent with rolling walker.*
   - *Chair: Independent with rolling walker.*
   - *Toilet: Independent with a three-in-one commode over the toilet.*
   - *Tub/shower: Minimum assistance with moderate cues with seat.*
   - *Car: Minimum assistance with minimum cues for technique.*

8. *Gait/functional mobility:* Independent ambulation with a rolling walker for 200 feet without resting. Stairs require supervision to assure foot clearance on the steps. She is not yet allowed to drive her car.

9. *Self-care (left dominant):*
   - *Feeding/equipment: Independent.*
   - *Bathing: Independent with upper body activities and stand/wash. Husband performs lower body bathing. Patient received a long-handled sponge and reacher in acute care.*
   - *Grooming: Independent.*
   - *Dressing: Independent except for lower body. Husband assists with all clothing below the knees. Patient also owns a long-handled shoehorn.*
   - *Toileting: Independent with the use of a three-in-one commode placed over the toilet.*
   - *Home management: Patient is assisting with meal preparation, seated. Using a walker basket. She demonstrates fair knowledge of bridging techniques.*
   - *Leisure/community: Currently she spends most of her time at home with friends/family coming to visit her.*

10. *ROM*: See Table 3-1.

11. *Strength*: See Table 3-2.

PATIENT GOALS

1. Independent self-care without equipment.
2. Independent transfers without a device, including showering.
3. Independent ambulation with or without a straight cane.
4. Home management tasks at an ambulatory level.
5. Return to volunteer position at the hospital.
6. Return to all other community activities.

EXERCISES FOR THE OT AND PT STUDENT

Case #15: Edna Marcusso

1. Using the Nagi scheme of disability, present the active pathology(ies), impairments, functional limitations, and disabilities for this case.

2. Do you think the patient's goals are realistic? Why or why not? If not, what strategies would you use to help the patient focus on more realistic goals?

3. Write an assessment and plan for the patient case(s) assigned. Include appropriate short-term and long-term goals.

4. Present a thorough plan of care for the case (ie, what specifically would you do with this patient and why?)

5. Design a treatment session lasting 30 minutes for this patient.

6. If both occupational and physical therapy were involved with this patient, what would you see as the role for each discipline to provide an appropriate, comprehensive treatment program? Consider the concepts of cotreatment and expert consultation in your answer.

7. Based upon the pathology that the patient exhibits and the individual impairments and functional limitations, do you think the patient will ever become totally "able" again? If not, which disabilities may remain?

8. What compensatory strategies might you teach the patient in this case?

9. What type(s) of DME (orthotic, prosthetic, or adaptive equipment) might you prescribe and why?

10. What would you propose as an appropriate treatment frequency and length of stay for this patient in your treatment setting? Provide the rationale for your answer.

11. What modifications would you have to make to the plan of care if you received insurance approval for only one-half of the time requested and the patient did not want to fund therapy privately?

12. Which portion(s) of the plan of care would you delegate to an assistant? Which portion(s) to an aide/tech? Provide your rationale for your answer.

13. For physical therapy students: Using the *Guidelines for Practice*, what would be your physical therapy diagnosis for this patient?

14. What environment(s) would you choose for implementing your treatment activities?

15. What activities would you use to address this patient's values?

16. Who is this patient? What roles and activities are important to her?

<u>Table 3-1</u>

Range of Motion

Left	Joint/Joint Complexes	Right	Comments
Neck			
¾ ROM	Flexion/extension	¾ ROM	
½ ROM	Rotation	½ ROM	
½ ROM	Lateral flexion	½ ROM	
Trunk			
½ ≈ ¾ ROM	Flexion/extension	½ ≈ ¾ ROM	
½ ≈ ¾ ROM	Rotation	½ ≈ ¾ ROM	
½ ≈ ¾ ROM	Lateral flexion	½ ≈ ¾ ROM	
½ ≈ ¾ ROM	Pelvic elevation	½ ≈ ¾ ROM	
Upper Extremities			
WFL	Scapular abd/add	WFL	She expresses discomfort at end ranges for both shoulders
WFL	Scapular elevation	WFL	
WFL	Shoulder flexion/extension	WFL	
WFL	Shoulder abd/add	WFL	
WFL	Shoulder IR/ER	WFL	
WFL	Shoulder horizontal abd/add	WFL	
WFL	Elbow flexion/extension	WFL	
WFL	Forearm pronation/supination	WFL	
WFL	Wrist flexion/extension	WFL	
WFL	MCP flexion/extension	WFL	
WFL	PIP flexion/extension	WFL	
WFL	DIP flexion/extension	WFL	
WFL	Finger abd/add	WFL	
WFL	Thumb MCP flexion/extension	WFL	
WFL	Thumb ICP flexion/extension	WFL	
WFL	Thumb abd/add	WFL	
WFL	Thumb opposition	WFL	
Lower Extremities			
WNL	SLR	60	
WNL	Hip flexion/extension	80 to -10	
WNL	Hip abd/add	25 to 0	

Table 3-1 continued

Left	Joint/Joint Complexes	Right	Comments
WNL	Hip IR/ER	0 to 30	
WNL	Knee flexion/extension	WNL	
WNL	Ankle plantar/dorsiflexion	WNL	
WNL	Foot eversion/inversion	WNL	
WNL	Great toe flexion/extension	WNL	
WNL	Toe MTP flexion/extension	WNL	
WNL	Toe IP flexion/extension	WNL	

abd = abduction; add = adduction; IR = internal rotation; ER = external rotation; MCP = metacarpophalangeal; PIP = proximal interphalangeal; DIP = distal interphalangeal; ICP = intermittent compression pump; WNL = within normal limits; SLR = straight leg raise.

Table 3-2

Manual Muscle Test

Left	Muscle/Muscle Group	Right	Comments
	Neck		
G-/G	Flexion/extension	G-/G	
F+	Rotation	F+	
G-	Lateral flexion	G-	
	Trunk		
WFL	Flexion/extension	WFL	
WFL	Rotation	WFL	
WFL	Lateral flexion	WFL	
WFL	Pelvic elevation	WFL	
	Upper Extremities		
WFL	Scapular abd/add	WFL	
WFL	Scapular elevation	WFL	
WFL	Shoulder flexion/extension	WFL	
WFL	Shoulder abd/add	WFL	
WFL	Shoulder IR/ER	WFL	
WFL	Shoulder horizontal abd/add	WFL	
WNL	Elbow flexion/extension	WNL	

Table 3-2 continued

Left	Muscle/Muscle Group	Right	Comments
WNL	Forearm pronation/supination	WNL	
WNL	Wrist flexion/extension	WNL	
WNL	MCP flexion/extension	WNL	
WNL	PIP flexion/extension	WNL	
WNL	DIP flexion/extension	WNL	
WNL	Finger abd/add	WNL	
WNL	Thumb MCP flexion/extension	WNL	
WNL	Thumb ICP flexion/extension	WNL	
WNL	Thumb abd/add	WNL	
WNL	Thumb opposition	WNL	
	Lower Extremities		
F+/G-	Hip flexion/extension	F-	
F+/G-	Hip abd/add	P+	
F+/G-	Hip IR/ER	F-	
G/N	Knee flexion/extension	G-/G	
G/N	Ankle plantar/dorsiflexion	G-/G	
G/N	Foot eversion/inversion	G-/G	
G/N	Great toe flexion/extension	G-/G	
G/N	Toe MTP flexion/extension	G-/G	
G/N	Toe IP flexion/extension	G-/G	

abd = abduction; add = adduction; IR = internal rotation; ER = external rotation; MCP = metacarpophalangeal; PIP = proximal interphalangeal; DIP = distal interphalangeal; ICP = intermittent compression pump; WNL = within normal limits; WFL = within functional limits; G = good (80%); G+ = good (90%); F = fair (50%); F+ = fair (60%); F- = fair (40%); P = poor (20%); P+ = poor (30%); P- = poor (10%).

EXERCISES FOR THE ASSISTANT STUDENT

CASE #15: EDNA MARCUSSO

1. Using the Nagi scheme of disability, present the active pathology(ies), impairments, functional limitations, and disabilities for this case.

2. Design a treatment session lasting 30 minutes for this patient.

3. If both occupational and physical therapy were involved with this patient, what would you see as the role for each discipline to provide an appropriate, comprehensive treatment program? Consider the concepts of cotreatment and expert consultation in your answer.

4. Based upon the pathology that the patient exhibits and the individual impairments and functional limitations, do you think the patient will ever become totally "able" again? If not, which disabilities may remain?

5. What compensatory strategies might you teach the patient in this case?

6. What type(s) of DME (orthotic, prosthetic, or adaptive equipment) might you prescribe and why?

7. Which portion(s) of the plan of care would you delegate to an aide/tech? Provide your rationale for your answer.

8. What environment(s) would you choose for implementing your treatment activities?

9. What activities would you use to address this patient's values?

10. Who is this patient? What roles and activities are important to her?

Juvenile Rheumatoid Arthritis

Laura Wadsworth is a 34-year-old woman with a 30-year history of juvenile rheumatoid arthritis (JRA). Her arthritis has progressed throughout the years, initially revealing itself as bilateral knee pain with erythema and edema, making functional mobility difficult. Since that time, Laura has undergone extensive orthopedic surgery to manage the joint deterioration from her JRA. These procedures include bilateral midtarsal joint fusions at age 20, right total knee replacement (TKR) at age 24, left TKR at age 26, left THR at age 28, right THR at age 30, which has since required two revision surgeries secondary to frequent dislocations, a right elbow arthroplasty at age 31 and, finally, second and third digit PIP and MCP arthroplasties on the right hand last year.

Throughout this time, she has lived independently in an apartment, which is architecturally barrier free and physically attached to her parent's four-bedroom home. Her mother does not work and has been available to Laura throughout her life to provide physical and emotional support whenever necessary. Laura is able to drive and has many friends with whom she spends her leisure time. She most enjoys relaxing over dinner in a nice restaurant and traveling when she is able.

She is unable to commit to a work schedule, either full- or part-time due to the frequent exacerbations of her disease but spends from 10 to 40 hours per week volunteering for the Arthritis Foundation. She does require an average of 8 weeks per year in which she does not work for the foundation due to surgeries, recovery, and vacation in the dry environment of the Southwest.

Laura seeks therapy services as an outpatient at this time, as she has noted increasing fatigue after completing her usual activities of daily living, complicated by difficulty with car and shower transfers and ambulation on level and stairs without an assistive device. She also reports a new onset of pain in her right shoulder, which is worse after overhead activities such as bathing and dressing.

She presents to you in the clinic with the following findings:

1. *Past medical history*: Insignificant for any issue other than her JRA diagnosis.

2. *Medications*: Ibuprofen and methotrexate.

3. *Cognition/perception*: Alert and oriented x 3. Without cognitive or perceptual deficit.

4. *Sensation*: Intact for all modalities on gross testing. Patient has occasional complaints of paresthesia in the median nerve distribution in the right wrist and hand, especially after prolonged computer use. Pain is a constant issue for this patient. She reports that despite her medications, her average daily pain is a 3 on a 1 to 10 scale, particularly in the hands, wrists, elbows, and now the right shoulder. Pain exacerbations are frequent and disabling and are accompanied by erythema and joint effusion in many of the joints of the upper and lower extremities. Her right hip, with frequent dislocations, is a constant source of pain as well.

5. *ROM*: See Table 3-3.

6. *Strength*: See Table 3-4.

7. *Balance*:
   - *Sitting: WNL*
   - *Stands with wide base of support. She can tolerate moderate challenges during static standing and can move throughout moderate active trunk excursions.*

8. *Mobility*:
   - *Bed mobility: Independent with increased effort to complete sit to supine and supine to sit due to lack of trunk rotation, and strength as well as pain.*

   Transfers:
   - *Sit → stand: Independent.*
   - *Bed ↔ chair: Independent.*
   - *Toilet: Independent.*
   - *Tub/shower: Minimum assistance.*
   - *Car: Minimum assistance with minimum cues for technique.*

9. *Gait*: Patient ambulates without a device for household mobility but uses a platform crutch in the left upper extremity for community/outdoor ambulation secondary to right lower extremity weakness and antalgic gait. She is independent in stair use with a rail and this assistive device. Gait analysis reveals decreased right stance time, limited heel strike, and push off with increased hip hike to clear the lower extremities. Trendelenburg's gait is also noted secondary to weakness in the hip abductors.

10. *Functional mobility*: Patient is able to perform all functional mobility tasks at an ambulatory level but does require the use of an assistive device. She is able to drive. Car transfers, especially to exit the vehicle, are particularly difficult secondary to weakness, lack of range of motion, and pain. She keeps a cell phone with her and when she arrives at her destination, she calls the individual whom she is visiting for minimal assistance if necessary. Therefore, she is not able to shop or perform other daily errands independently but waits until her mother or a friend has time to go with her to accomplish these tasks. In addition, she requires supervision for shower transfers despite the availability of a grab bar in the shower. She is anxious during shower transfers, as hiking and lifting her lower extremities into the tub requires as much strength as she has and is quite painful.

Table 3-3

Transfers

Left	Joint/Joint Complexes	Right	Comments
	Neck		
½ range	Flexion/extension	½ range	
½ range	Rotation	½ range	
½ range	Lateral flexion	½ range	
	Trunk		
½ range	Flexion/extension	½ range	
½ range	Rotation	½ range	
½ range	Lateral flexion	½ range	
¾ range	Pelvic elevation	¾ range	
	Upper Extremities		
Mod↓	Scapular abd/add	Mod↓	
Mod↓	Scapular elevation	Mod↓	
120/10 degrees	Shoulder flexion/extension	90/10 degrees	
110/0 degrees	Shoulder abd/add	88/0 degrees	
WNL/75 degrees	Shoulder IR/ER	WNL/70 degrees	
WNL	Shoulder horizontal abd/add	WNL	
100/-20 degrees	Elbow flexion/extension	95/-20 degrees	
WNL	Forearm pronation/supination	WNL	
Mod↓	Wrist flexion/extension	Mod↓	
Mod/sev↓	MCP flexion/extension	Mod/sev↓	
Mod/sev↓	PIP flexion/extension	Mod/sev↓	
Mod/sev↓	DIP flexion/extension	Mod/sev↓	
Mod/sev↓	Finger abd/add	Mod/sev↓	
Mod/sev↓	Thumb MCP flexion/extension	Mod/sev↓	
Mod/sev↓	Thumb ICP flexion/extension	Mod/sev↓	
Mod/sev↓	Thumb abd/add	Mod/sev↓	
Mod/sev↓	Thumb opposition	Mod/sev↓	
	Lower Extremities		
45 degrees	SLR	40 degrees	
90/10 degrees	Hip flexion/extension	85/5 degrees	
30/0 degrees	Hip abd/add	28/0 degrees	

Table 3-3 continued

Left	Joint/Joint Complexes	Right	Comments
0/20 degrees	Hip IR/ER	0/20 degrees	
90/0 degrees	Knee flexion/extension	85/-5 degrees	Tested in sitting
20/0 degrees	Ankle plantar/dorsiflexion	20/0 degrees	
Sev ↓	Foot eversion/inversion	Sev ↓	Secondary to fusion
Mod ↓	Great toe flexion/extension	Mod ↓	
Mod ↓	Toe MTP flexion/extension	Mod ↓	
Mod ↓	Toe IP flexion/extension	Mod ↓	

Mod ↓ = moderate decrease; min ↓ = minimal decrease; sev ↓ = severe decrease; abd = abduction; add = adduction; IR = internal rotation; ER = external rotation; MCP = metacarpophalangeal; PIP = proximal interphalangeal; DIP = distal interphalangeal; ICP = intermittent compression pump; WNL = within normal limits; WFL = within functional limits; SLR = straight leg raise.

Table 3-4

Manual Muscle Test

Left	Muscle/Muscle Group	Right	Comments
	Neck		
			All neck, trunk, and upper extremity muscles tested functionally secondary to joint deformity and/or pain
≥ F	Flexion/extension	≥ F	
≥ F	Rotation	≥ F	
≥ F	Lateral flexion	≥ F	
	Trunk		
≥ P+/F-	Flexion/extension	≥ P+/F-	
≥ P+/F-	Rotation	≥ P+/F-	
≥ P+/F-	Lateral flexion	≥ P+/F-	
F	Pelvic elevation	F	
	Upper Extremities		
F	Scapular abd/add	F	
F	Scapular elevation	F	
≥ F+	Shoulder flexion/extension	≥ F+	
≥ F+	Shoulder abd/add	≥ F+	

<u>Table 3-4 continued</u>

Left	Muscle/Muscle Group	Right	Comments
≥ F+	Shoulder IR/ER	≥ F+	
≥ F+	Shoulder horizontal abd/add	≥ F+	
F+/G-	Elbow flexion/extension	F+/G-	
≥ F	Forearm pronation/supination	≥ F	
F	Wrist flexion/extension	≥ F	
≥ F	MCP flexion/extension	≥ F	
≥ F	PIP flexion/extension	≥ F	
≥ F	DIP flexion/extension	≥ F	
≥ F	Finger abd/add	≥ F	
≥ F	Thumb MCP flexion/extension	≥ F	
≥ F	Thumb ICP flexion/extension	≥ F	
≥ F	Thumb abd/add	≥ F	
≥ F	Thumb opposition	≥ F	
	Lower Extremities		
F+/P+	Hip flexion/extension	F/P	
P+/P+	Hip abd/add	P/P	
F-/F-	Hip IR/ER	F-/F-	
F/F	Knee flexion/extension	F/F	Tested in sitting
P+/F	Ankle plantar/dorsiflexion	P+/F	
NT	Foot eversion/inversion	NT	Secondary to fusion
≥ F	Great toe flexion/extension	≥ F	Tested functionally secondary to joint deformity
≥ F	Toe MTP flexion/extension	≥ F	
≥ F	Toe IP flexion/extension	≥ F	

abd = abduction; add = adduction; IR = internal rotation; ER = external rotation; MCP = metacarpophalangeal; PIP = proximal interphalangeal; DIP = distal interphalangeal; ICP = intermittent oppression pump; WNL = within normal limits; WFL = within functional limits; G = good (80%); G+ = good (90%); F = fair (50%); F+ = fair (60%); F- = fair (40%); P = poor (20%); P+ = poor (30%); P- = poor (10%).

11. *Self-care*: Patient is independent with feeding, toileting, sponge bathing, grooming, and dressing with adaptive equipment to compensate for lack of hand function, lower extremity strength, and range of motion deficits and pain. She is having increased difficulty with upper extremity (UE) dressing due to new complaints of shoulder immobility. She can feed herself independently using light weight dinnerware with built-up handles on the utensils.

12. *Home management*: Patient is unable to lift any weight greater than 5 lbs. She therefore needs assistance for heavy housework and has a housekeeper once a week to accomplish heavy cleaning and laundry. The patient is able to perform light tasks such as dusting and washing the dishes. She prepares meals for herself independently with the use of adaptive equipment. She manages her finances independently.

PATIENT GOALS

1. Independent functional transfers (car and shower).
2. Independent gait without an assistive device for home and community-level function.
3. Minimize fatigue and pain to improve ability to perform all ADL, especially her right UE.

EXERCISES FOR THE OT AND PT STUDENT

Case #16: Laura Wadsworth

1. Using the Nagi scheme of disability, present the active pathology(ies), impairments, functional limitations, and disabilities for this case.

2. Do you think the patient's goals are realistic? Why or why not? If not, what strategies would you use to help the patient focus on more realistic goals?

3. Write an assessment and plan for the patient case(s) assigned. Include appropriate short-term and long-term goals.

4. Present a thorough plan of care for the case (ie, what specifically would you do with this patient and why?)

5. Design a treatment session lasting 30 minutes for this patient.

6. If both occupational and physical therapy were involved with this patient, what would you see as the role for each discipline to provide an appropriate, comprehensive treatment program? Consider the concepts of cotreatment and expert consultation in your answer.

7. Based upon the pathology that the patient exhibits and the individual impairments and functional limitations, do you think the patient will ever become totally "able" again? If not, which disabilities may remain?

8. What compensatory strategies might you teach the patient in this case?

9. What type(s) of DME (orthotic, prosthetic, or adaptive equipment) might you prescribe and why?

10. What would you propose as an appropriate treatment frequency and length of stay for this patient in your treatment setting? Provide the rationale for your answer.

11. What modifications would you have to make to the plan of care if you received insurance approval for only one-half of the time requested and the patient did not to fund therapy privately?

12. Which portion(s) of the plan of care would you delegate to an assistant? Which portion(s) to an aide/tech? Provide your rationale for your answer.

13. For physical therapy students: Using the *Guidelines for Practice*, what would be your physical therapy diagnosis for this patient?

14. What environment(s) would you choose for implementing your treatment activities?

15. What activities would you use to address this patient's values?

16. Who is this patient? What roles and activities are important to her?

EXERCISES FOR THE ASSISTANT STUDENT

Case #16: Laura Wadsworth

1. Using the Nagi scheme of disability, present the active pathology(ies), impairments, functional limitations, and disabilities for this case.

2. Design a treatment session lasting 30 minutes for this patient.

3. If both occupational and physical therapy were involved with this patient, what would you see as the role for each discipline to provide an appropriate, comprehensive treatment program? Consider the concepts of cotreatment and expert consultation in your answer.

4. Based upon the pathology that the patient exhibits and the individual impairments and functional limitations, do you think the patient will ever become totally "able" again? If not, which disabilities may remain?

5. What compensatory strategies might you teach the patient in this case?

6. What type(s) of DME (orthotic, prosthetic, or adaptive equipment) might you prescribe and why?

7. Which portion(s) of the plan of care would you delegate to an aide/tech? Provide your rationale for your answer.

8. What environment(s) would you choose for implementing your treatment activities?

9. What activities would you use to address this patient's values?

10. Who is this patient? What roles and activities are important to her?

Ankylosing Spondylitis

Howard Longo was a typical 35-year-old man, a married software engineer with three children—2, 8, and 11 years of age—when he began to have frequent stiffness in his low back upon arising each morning and pain in his right hip after prolonged high-impact activities, such as during his daily 5-mile walk. After 2 months of persistent symptoms, he sought out medical care with the urging of his wife. His internist referred him to a rheumatologist, as some type of arthritis was suspected. The rheumatologist confirmed that indeed Howard did have ankylosing spondylitis, a systemic type of rheumatologic disease. At that time, he was advised to remain as active as possible and was prescribed non-steroidal anti-inflammatory drugs to reduce his pain and stiffness.

Howard was concerned about his diagnosis at the time but did not choose to learn more about it and, as his pain and stiffness were under control, he continued his life as usual. For Howard this meant that he worked 45 to 60 hours per week, managed his son's hockey team, took his daughter to swimming lessons, and transported his youngest son to daycare each day. His wife worked full-time as a manager of a local bookstore. She was also very active with the children, supporting their efforts in both school and recreational endeavors. She was an active member of the PTA and in the spring coached her daughter's T-ball team. The family lives in a two-story single family home with three steps to enter and one flight to the second floor bedroom and bathroom that Howard shares with his wife. The children each have their own room and share a bathroom on the second floor. There is a half bath on the first floor off the kitchen. They have a housekeeper to manage basic cleaning and household tasks once a week.

Two years later, his disease had progressed significantly. He was now taking prednisone in addition to his nonsteroidal anti-inflammatory drugs to decrease the steadily worsening symptoms of pain and stiffness that had now progressed into his entire back, neck, and pelvis. By the time he reached 40, his disease had progressed to the point where he demonstrated significant deficits in strength, lower extremity range of motion, posture, and endurance. These issues, in combination with persistent pain, resulted in loss of function for Howard. He was no longer able to walk more than 1 mile for exercise and was having great difficulty attending hockey games due to the cold temperature of the rink and the length of time he needed to be on his feet. He could no longer sit for more than 1 hour without debilitating stiffness in his back, hips, and pelvic areas, making it difficult for him to complete his job duties. In addition, he was having difficulty keeping up with the demands of his family life, which resulted in his wife having to manage more of the home and childcare responsibilities. Finally, he was having trouble using the stairs to access his bedroom and bathroom.

When he had his last rheumatology appointment, the doctor stated that his right hip had deteriorated to the point where the only alternative for Howard was to have a total hip replacement in order to regain a relatively pain free and active lifestyle. Howard was reluctant to have this surgery, as he was concerned that if he had a total hip replacement at the age of 40 he would need to have multiple revisions in the future (the doctor had told him that the replacement "only lasts so long perhaps 10 to 15 years at best"). Howard was not comfortable thinking of himself as disabled and was particularly anxious about the idea of having surgery. He was quite upset about the fact that more surgery may be necessary in his future. He decided to try a course of physical and occupational therapy to see what these services may offer him prior to deciding to have a total hip replacement.

He presents to you in the clinic with the following findings:

1. *Past medical history*: Right anterior cruciate ligament (ACL) repair after a skiing injury 12 years ago. Mild HTN diagnosed 2 years ago; average resting BP range is 146/98 to 150/100.

2. *Medications*: Tenormin, prednisone, ibuprofen.

3. *Cognition/perception*: Alert and oriented x3. Without cognitive or perceptual deficit.

4. *ROM*: See Table 3-5.

5. *Strength*: See Table 3-6.

6. *Neurology*: Intact for sensation. Without abnormal muscle tone.

7. *Balance*: Patient is only able to move through moderate active trunk excursions due to limited ROM and can take only moderate external perturbations (pushes) without loss of balance.

8. *Pain*: At rest this patient's primary complaint is the development of stiffness throughout his trunk, which makes mobility initiation difficult. Pain in his bilateral hips is noted primarily with activities such as lifting and carrying or prolonged standing statically and dynamically. He rates his pain as a 4 on a 1 to 10 scale in his left hip and 6 on a 1 to 10 scale in his right hip at these times.

9. *Mobility*:
   * *Bed mobility: Upon evaluation the patient is able to use compensatory strategies to perform supine to sit on a firm mat; however, this patient reports needing the assistance of his wife 3 of 7 days to attain sitting from supine in bed.*
   * *Rolling: Independent with log roll side to side and side to prone.*
   * *Bridging: Able to complete half bridge independently with limits secondary to ROM deficiency.*
   * *Supine ↔ sit: Minimum assist supine to sit; independent sit to supine.*
   * *Equipment: None used presently.*
   * *Transfers: Patient requires minimum assistance to attain standing from a low chair without arms or from the floor. Patient is unable to bend down and pick up an object greater than 25 lbs from the floor without minimal assistance.*
   * *Sit → stand: Ranges from minimum assistance to independent depending upon the transfer surface.*
   * *Bed ↔ chair: Independent.*
   * *Toilet: Independent with a raised toilet seat.*
   * *Tub/shower: Minimum assistance.*
   * *Car: Independent with patient using UE on seat back and door to push up for exiting the car.*

10. *Gait*: Patient is completely independent in ambulation but is noting increased pain with his endurance exercise of walking one-half mile three times per week. He dem-

Table 3-5

Range of Motion

Left	Joint/Joint Complexes	Right	Comments
	Neck		
¾ range	Flexion/extension	¾ range	
½ range	Rotation	½ range	
½ range	Lateral flexion	½ range	
	Trunk		
¼ to ½ range	Flexion/extension	¼ to ½ range	
½ range	Rotation	½ range	
½ range	Lateral flexion	½ range	
½ range	Pelvic elevation	½ range	
	Upper Extremities		
WNL	Scapular abd/add	WNL	
WNL	Scapular elevation	WNL	
WNL	Shoulder flexion/extension	WNL	
WNL	Shoulder abd/add	WNL	
WNL	Shoulder IR/ER	WNL	
WNL	Shoulder horizontal abd/add	WNL	
WNL	Elbow flexion/extension	WNL	
WNL	Forearm pronation/supination	WNL	
WNL	Wrist flexion/extension	WNL	
WNL	MCP flexion/extension	WNL	
WNL	PIP flexion/extension	WNL	
WNL	DIP flexion/extension	WNL	
WNL	Finger abd/add	WNL	
WNL	Thumb MCP flexion/extension	WNL	
WNL	Thumb ICP flexion/extension	WNL	
WNL	Thumb abd/add	WNL	
WNL	Thumb opposition	WNL	
	Lower Extremities		
40 degrees	SLR	40 degrees	
95/0 degrees	Hip flexion/extension	80/-10 degrees	
30/10 degrees	Hip abd/add	30/10 degrees	

Table 3-5 continued

Left	Joint/Joint Complexes	Right	Comments
WNL	Hip IR/ER	WNL	
WNL	Knee flexion/extension	90/-5 degrees	
WNL	Ankle plantar/dorsiflexion	WNL	
WNL	Foot eversion/inversion	WNL	
WNL	Great toe flexion/extension	WNL	
WNL	Toe MTP flexion/extension	WNL	
WNL	Toe IP flexion/extension	WNL	

abd = abduction; add = adduction; IR = internal rotation; ER = external rotation; MCP = metacarpophalangeal; PIP = proximal interphalangeal; DIP = distal interphalangeal; ICP = intermittent compression pump; WNL = within normal limits; WFL = within functional limits; SLR = straight leg raise.

Table 3-6

Manual Muscle Test

Left	Muscle/Muscle Group	Right	Comments
	Neck		
F/F	Flexion/extension	F/F	Tested functionally
F/F	Rotation	F/F	Tested functionally
F/F	Lateral flexion	F/F	Tested functionally
	Trunk		
P+/F-	Flexion/extension	P+/F-	Tested functionally
P+	Rotation	P+	Tested functionally
P+	Lateral flexion	P+	Tested functionally
F	Pelvic elevation	F-	Tested functionally
	Upper Extremities		
WNL	Scapular abd/add	WNL	
WNL	Scapular elevation	WNL	
WNL	Shoulder flexion/extension	WNL	
WNL	Shoulder abd/add	WNL	
WNL	Shoulder IR/ER	WNL	
WNL	Shoulder horizontal abd/add	WNL	

Table 3-6 continued

Left	Muscle/Muscle Group	Right	Comments
WNL	Elbow flexion/extension	WNL	
WNL	Forearm pronation/supination	WNL	
WNL	Wrist flexion/extension	WNL	
WNL	MCP flexion/extension	WNL	
WNL	PIP flexion/extension	WNL	
WNL	DIP flexion/extension	WNL	
WNL	Finger abd/add	WNL	
WNL	Thumb MCP flexion/extension	WNL	
WNL	Thumb ICP flexion/extension	WNL	
WNL	Thumb abd/add	WNL	
WNL	Thumb opposition	WNL	
	Lower Extremities		
G/F-	Hip flexion/extension	F/P+	Right hip MMT with minimum complaints of pain
F/F	Hip abd/add	P+/P+	
F/F	Hip IR/ER	F-/F-	
G-/G	Knee flexion/extension	F+/G-	
WNL	Ankle plantar/dorsiflexion	WNL	
WNL	Foot eversion/inversion	WNL	
WNL	Great toe flexion/extension	WNL	
WNL	Toe MTP flexion/extension	WNL	
WNL	Toe IP flexion/extension	WNL	

abd = abduction; add = adduction; IR = internal rotation; ER = external rotation; MCP = metacarpophalangeal; PIP = proximal interphalangeal; DIP = distal interphalangeal; ICP = intermittent compression pump; WNL = within normal limits; WFL = within functional limits; G = good (80%); G+ = good (90%); F = fair (50%); F+ = fair (60%); F- = fair (40%); P = poor (20%); P+ = poor (30%); P- = poor (10%).

onstrates decreased stance time on the RLE and forward flexion at the hips and trunk. His trunk rotation is poor. Cadence is slow. Stair climbing is strenuous and painful, however, the patient can ascend and descend one flight of stairs with rail.

11. *Functional mobility*: Patient is able to complete all job duties independently but with great effort and increased pain and stiffness, especially with prolonged sitting at his computer terminal. He enjoys a tub bath one to two times per week but requires occasional minimum assistance to complete tub transfers.

12. *Self-care*: Patient is independent in all self-care activities with the exception of tub transfers. He uses a long-handled shoe horn to don/doff shoes independently. He does report having significant difficulty donning and doffing socks and goes without wearing them whenever possible. He states that his wife provides occasional minimum assistance to don/doff socks when his pain and stiffness are particularly severe. He requires moderate assistance to don/doff his pants.

- *Home management: Patient is not responsible for any of the basic home care and management tasks. He reports that although he would like to do all of the basic maintenance work at home, he often relies on hired help to perform these tasks due to his pain, stiffness, and lack of strength and endurance.*

PATIENT GOALS

1. Independent bed mobility 7 of 7 days at home.

2. Independent transfers to and from all surfaces.

3. Ability to complete job duties with less pain and stiffness.

4. Independent ability to exercise on a daily basis with less pain.

5. Independent gait on level and stairs for home and community functions with minimal pain.

6. Independent self-care including the ability to bathe in the tub and dress his lower body.

EXERCISES FOR THE OT AND PT STUDENT

Case #17: Howard Longo

1. Using the Nagi scheme of disability, present the active pathology(ies), impairments, functional limitations, and disabilities for this case.

2. Do you think the patient's goals are realistic? Why or why not? If not, what strategies would you use to help the patient focus on more realistic goals?

3. Write an assessment and plan for the patient case(s) assigned. Include appropriate short-term and long-term goals.

4. Present a thorough plan of care for the case (ie, what specifically would you do with this patient and why?)

5. Design a treatment session lasting 30 minutes for this patient.

6. If both occupational and physical therapy were involved with this patient, what would you see as the role for each discipline to provide an appropriate, comprehensive treatment program? Consider the concepts of cotreatment and expert consultation in your answer.

7. Based upon the pathology that the patient exhibits and the individual impairments and functional limitations, do you think the patient will ever become totally "able" again? If not, which disabilities may remain?

8. What compensatory strategies might you teach the patient in this case?

9. What type(s) of DME (orthotic, prosthetic, or adaptive equipment) might you prescribe and why?

10. What would you propose as an appropriate treatment frequency and length of stay for this patient in your treatment setting? Provide the rationale for your answer.

11. What modifications would you have to make to the plan of care if you received insurance approval for only one-half of the time requested and the patient did not want to fund therapy privately?

12. Which portion(s) of the plan of care would you delegate to an assistant? Which portion(s) to an aide/tech? Provide your rationale for your answer.

13. For physical therapy students: Using the *Guidelines for Practice*, what would be your physical therapy diagnosis for this patient?

14. What environment(s) would you choose for implementing your treatment activities?

15. What activities would you use to address this patient's values?

16. Who is this patient? What roles and activities are important to him?

EXERCISES FOR THE ASSISTANT STUDENT

Case #17: Howard Longo

1. Using the Nagi scheme of disability, present the active pathology(ies), impairments, functional limitations, and disabilities for this case.

2. Design a treatment session lasting 30 minutes for this patient.

3. If both occupational and physical therapy were involved with this patient, what would you see as the role for each discipline to provide an appropriate, comprehensive treatment program? Consider the concepts of cotreatment and expert consultation in your answer.

4. Based upon the pathology that the patient exhibits and the individual impairments and functional limitations, do you think the patient will ever become totally "able" again? If not, which disabilities may remain?

5. What compensatory strategies might you teach the patient in this case?

6. What type(s) of DME (orthotic, prosthetic, or adaptive equipment) might you prescribe and why?

7. Which portion(s) of the plan of care would you delegate to an aide/tech? Provide your rationale for your answer.

8. What environment (s) would you choose for implementing your treatment activities?

9. What activities would you use to address this patient's values?

10. Who is this patient? What roles and activities are important to him?

ONCOLOGY

Breast Cancer

Melinda Wells, age 57, is the mother of two adult daughters and the grandmother of three. She is divorced and remarried at the age of 45. Her current husband is 20 years her senior and is retired. She feels lucky; both daughters live nearby and are able to visit frequently. Her relationship with her husband is peripheral to her relationships with her daughters.

Upon her husband's retirement, they sold their home and bought a new home in a development. The townhouse has two floors with a half-bathroom and a large open space on the first floor. The second floor has two bedrooms and a full standard bathroom. There are four railed steps up to the front porch.

During a routine physical examination, Mrs. Wells was informed of a lump in her left breast. Although she was quite frightened, she prayed everything would run its course and that all would be fine. It seemed as if her world suddenly went topsy-turvy. Things seemed surreal and before she knew it, she had her left breast removed along with its associated lymph nodes.

Her husband felt removed from the picture. He was uncertain as to how to speak to Melinda. Moreover, Melinda did not know what to say. Her daughters hovered and were frequently sobbing. All Melinda knew is that she wanted to be at home and make this bad dream go away.

During her recovery, she received radiation and therapy. Her left arm movements were limited. She had severe and recurrent problems with edema in her LUE. She received pressure garments and the therapist utilized a pump on the extremity. She was diagnosed with lymphedema. The arm felt heavy and ready to burst. Her balance was also disturbed by the extra weight on one side. She was discharged to her home with orders to receive therapy at home. She plans to continue to travel 25 miles each way to receive chemotherapy.

At home, she has remained in a reclining chair because of her limited mobility and increased pain upon standing due to gravity's effects on her LUE. She has no DME and seems depressed and immobilized by her current situation.

She has therapy orders for evaluation and treatment at home. The results of her initial evaluation are as follows:

1. *Perception/cognition*: WNL

2. *Sensation/pain*: Intact. However, hypersensitivity is present throughout LUE. Patient complains of pulling and bursting feeling of LUE.

3. *Skin/edema*: Marked deep pitting edema noted throughout LUE. Wrist measures 24 cm; elbow 32 cm; axillary area 44 cm.

4. *Balance*: Supported static sit is normal when LUE is slung/supported. Marked difficulty for control during dynamic sit due to LUE weight. Patient can be easily displaced in standing due to LUE and patient discomfort.

5. *Mobility:*
Bed mobility:

- *Rolling: Patient refuses to lie in bed secondary to discomfort and fear of not being able to get up.*
- *Bridging: Patient refuses to lie in bed secondary to discomfort and fear of not being able to get up.*
- *Supine ↔ sit: Patient refuses to lie in bed secondary to discomfort and fear of not being able to get up.*
- *Equipment: Patient refuses to lie in bed secondary to discomfort and fear of not being able to get up.*

Transfers:

- *Sit → stand: Minimum assistance to support left trunk/extremity.*
- *Bed: NT.*

- *Chair* ↔ *stand: Same as sit to stand.*
- *Toilet* ↔ *stand: Moderate assistance to support left trunk/extremity.*
- *Tub/shower: NT due to patient's fear of falling (no equipment is available).*
- *Car: NT.*

6. *Gait/functional mobility*: Ambulates with LUE in sling. Ambulates with minimum to moderate support of one (depends on fatigue and distance). She is able to ambulate within her home. There is a moderate increase in her base of support with minimal forward flexion at the hips.

7. *Self-care (right dominant)*

- *Feeding/equipment: All food must be cut up. Self feeds but reports having a poor appetite. Would like to cut her own food because, "Not feeding yourself makes you feel really helpless."*
- *Bathing: Maximum assistance for both upper and lower body as patient sits on the toilet to bathe. The sink is located next to toilet. Needs assistance for stand/wash. Also, complains of fatigue. Patient reports not having much motivation to care for herself.*
- *Grooming: After set-up, brushes her teeth and combs her hair.*
- *Dressing: Maximum assistance to don dress with snaps down the front. Dependent for footwear. Prefers not to wear underwear.*
- *Toileting: Completes hygiene by leaning against the wall for support.*
- *Home management: Dependent.*
- *Leisure/community: Listens to TV and has family with her at most times. Reports not sleeping well at night.*

8. *ROM*: See Table 4-1.

9. *Strength*: See Table 4-2.

PATIENT GOALS

1. LUE edema control.
2. Independent toileting.
3. Ability to recline in bed.
4. Independent ambulation in her home.
5. Supervised ability to shower.
6. Ability to use LUE in bilateral tasks.

EXERCISES FOR THE OT AND PT STUDENT

Case #18: Melinda Wells

1. Using the Nagi scheme of disability, present the active pathology(ies), impairments, functional limitations, and disabilities for this case.

2. Do you think the patient's goals are realistic? Why or why not? If not, what strategies would you use to help the patient focus on more realistic goals?

3. Write an assessment and plan for the patient case(s) assigned. Include appropriate short-term and long-term goals.

4. Present a thorough plan of care for the case (ie, what specifically would you do with this patient and why?).

5. Design a treatment session lasting 30 minutes for this patient.

6. If both occupational and physical therapy were involved with this patient, what would you see as the role for each discipline to provide an appropriate, comprehensive treatment program? Consider the concepts of cotreatment and expert consultation in your answer.

7. Based upon the pathology that the patient exhibits and the individual impairments and functional limitations, do you think the patient will ever become totally "able" again? If not, which disabilities may remain?

8. What compensatory strategies might you teach the patient in this case?

9. What type(s) of DME (orthotic, prosthetic, or adaptive equipment) might you prescribe and why?

10. What would you propose as an appropriate treatment frequency and length of stay for this patient in your treatment setting? Provide the rationale for your answer.

11. What modifications would you have to make to the plan of care if you received insurance approval for only one-half of the time requested and the patient did not want to fund therapy privately?

12. Which portion(s) of the plan of care would you delegate to an assistant? Which portion(s) to an aide/tech? Provide your rationale for your answer.

13. For physical therapy students: Using the *Guidelines for Practice*, what would be your physical therapy diagnosis for this patient?

14. What environment(s) would you choose for implementing your treatment activities?

15. What activities would you use to address this patient's values?

16. Who is this patient? What roles and activities are important to her?

17. What community supports could you use for this home care patient to address her need for psychosocial support?

EXERCISES FOR THE ASSISTANT STUDENT

Case #18: Melinda Wells

1. Using the Nagi scheme of disability, present the active pathology(ies), impairments, functional limitations, and disabilities for this case.

<u>Table 4-1</u>

Range of Motion

Left	Joint/Joint Complexes	Right	Comments
	Neck		
WFL	Flexion/extension	WNL	
WFL	Rotation	WNL	
WFL	Lateral flexion	WNL	
	Trunk		
WFL	Flexion/extension	WNL	
WFL	Rotation	WNL	
WFL	Lateral flexion	WNL	
WFL	Pelvic elevation	WNL	
	Upper Extremities		
WFL	Scapular abd/add	WNL	
WFL	Scapular elevation	WNL	
≈ 80/0	Shoulder flexion/extension	WNL	
≈ 60/full	Shoulder abd/add	WNL	
Full/≈ 30	Shoulder IR/ER	WNL	
NT	Shoulder horizontal abd/add	WNL	
≈ 3/4	Elbow flexion/extension	WNL	
WFL	Forearm pronation/supination	WNL	
≈ 3/4	Wrist flexion/extension	WNL	
≈ 3/4	MCP flexion/extension	WNL	
≈ 3/4	PIP flexion/extension	WNL	
≈ 3/4	DIP flexion/extension	WNL	
≈ 3/4	Finger abd/add	WNL	
≈ 3/4	Thumb MCP flexion/extension	WNL	
≈ 3/4	Thumb ICP flexion/extension	WNL	
≈ 3/4	Thumb abd/add	WNL	
≈ 3/4	Thumb opposition	WNL	
	Lower Extremities		
WNL	SLR	WNL	
WNL	Hip flexion/extension	WNL	
WNL	Hip abd/add	WNL	

Table 4-1 continued

Left	Joint/Joint Complexes	Right	Comments
WNL	Hip IR/ER	WNL	
WNL	Knee flexion/extension	WNL	
WNL	Ankle plantar/dorsiflexion	WNL	
WNL	Foot eversion/inversion	WNL	
WNL	Great toe flexion/extension	WNL	
WNL	Toe MTP flexion/extension	WNL	
WNL	Toe IP flexion/extension	WNL	

abd = abduction; add = adduction; IR = internal rotation; ER = external rotation; MCP = metacarpophalangeal; PIP = proximal interphalangeal; DIP = distal interphalangeal; ICP = intermittent compression pump; WNL = within normal limits; SLR = straight leg raise; ≈ = approximately.

Table 4-2

Manual Muscle Test

Left	Muscle/Muscle Group	Right	Comments
	Neck		
G-	Flexion/extension	Normal	
G-	Rotation	Normal	
G-	Lateral flexion	Normal	
	Trunk		
G-	Flexion/extension	Normal	
G-	Rotation	Normal	
G-	Lateral flexion	Normal	
G-	Pelvic elevation	Normal	
	Upper Extremities		
G-	Scapular abd/add	Normal	LUE is able to take resistance against gravity
G-	Scapular elevation	Normal	
G-	Shoulder flexion/extension	Normal	
G-	Shoulder abd/add	Normal	
G-	Shoulder IR/ER	Normal	
G-	Shoulder horizontal abd/add	Normal	

Table 4-2 continued

Left	Muscle/Muscle Group	Right	Comments
G-	Elbow flexion/extension	Normal	
G-	Forearm pronation/supination	Normal	
G-	Wrist flexion/extension	Normal	
G-	MCP flexion/extension	Normal	Has gross grasp and pinch difficulty with fine motor tasks
G-	PIP flexion/extension	Normal	
G-	DIP flexion/extension	Normal	
G-	Finger abd/add	Normal	
G-	Thumb MCP flexion/extension	Normal	
G-	Thumb ICP flexion/extension	Normal	
G-	Thumb abd/add	Normal	
G-	Thumb opposition	Normal	
	Lower Extremities		
Normal	Hip flexion/extension	Normal	
Normal	Hip abd/add	Normal	
Normal	Hip IR/ER	Normal	
Normal	Knee flexion/extension	Normal	
Normal	Ankle plantar/dorsiflexion	Normal	
Normal	Foot eversion/inversion	Normal	
Normal	Great toe flexion/extension	Normal	
Normal	Toe MTP flexion/extension	Normal	
Normal	Toe IP flexion/extension	Normal	

abd = abduction; add = adduction; IR = internal rotation; ER = external rotation; MCP = metacarpophalangeal; PIP = proximal interphalangeal; DIP = distal interphalangeal; ICP = intermittent compression pump; WNL = within normal limits; WFL = within functional limits; G = good (80%); G+ = good (90%); F = fair (50%); F+ = fair (60%); F- = fair (40%); P = poor (20%); P+ = poor (30%); P- = poor (10%).

2. Design a treatment session lasting 30 minutes for this patient.

3. If both occupational and physical therapy were involved with this patient, what would you see as the role for each discipline to provide an appropriate, comprehensive treatment program? Consider the concepts of cotreatment and expert consultation in your answer.

4. Based upon the pathology that the patient exhibits and the individual impairments and functional limitations, do you think the patient will ever become totally "able" again? If not, which disabilities may remain?

5. What compensatory strategies might you teach the patient in this case?

6. What type(s) of DME (orthotic, prosthetic, or adaptive equipment) might you prescribe and why?

7. Which portion(s) of the plan of care would you delegate to an aide/tech? Provide your rationale for your answer.

8. What environment(s) would you choose for implementing your treatment activities?

9. What activities would you use to address this patient's values?

10. Who is this patient? What roles and activities are important to her?

11. What community supports could you use for this home care patient to address her need for psychosocial support?

Colon Cancer

Sonya Wellfleet was a typical 48-year-old woman who lived with her husband and their two teenage children in a single family suburban home when she began to have frequent episodes of abdominal pain with diarrhea. Initially she managed her symptoms with over-the-counter antidiarrhea medication, which helped to some extent. At that time, she continued on with her busy lifestyle of working full-time as an administrative assistant and fulfilling her role as wife and mother. Her children kept her especially busy, as both played basketball and soccer for their high school teams. One child also played saxophone in the jazz band, while the other had a 10-hour-a-week job at the local grocery store. All of these activities required Sonya to be available to transport the children to and from activities, as her husband worked long hours as the CFO of a large equipment corporation. She did have weekly help with the housekeeping responsibilities from a cleaning agency but needed to perform daily clean-up and pick-up routines that busy families require. Also, she did the grocery shopping for the family.

She began to become concerned 2 months later when the episodes of abdominal pain and diarrhea became more regular and she noticed that she had lost 10 pounds unexpectedly during this time. At that time she made an appointment with her internist. Her physician did a thorough physical examination including a digital rectal examination, bloodwork, and stool examination for occult blood. When the bloodwork came back positive for anemia and there was occult blood in the stool, her physician became concerned as well. Sonya had a sigmoidoscopy, which revealed polyps in the colon. A biopsy confirmed the diagnosis of colon cancer. All other medical tests were negative for metastatic disease at that time. She underwent a colectomy within 2 weeks of the diagnosis and began a course of chemotherapy. Recovery from the surgery went well for Sonya and she tolerated the chemotherapy reasonably well, although she did take a medical leave of absence from work during this time.

Six months later, Sonya began to feel unusually fatigued with normal activities of daily living and noticed that she was having some back pain and abdominal cramps. She once again sought out medical consult and, unfortunately, found out that the cancer had returned with metastases to the liver and lungs. Her functional status has rapidly declined and she is referred to your skilled nursing facility for 2 weeks of inpatient rehabilitation to recover maximum functional status with compensatory strategies as needed. Her primary goal is to return home and be with her family and function as independently as possible, for as long as possible.

She presents to you in the clinic with the following findings:

1. *Significant PMH*: Obesity, hypercholesteremia, two cesarean births, s/p colectomy. Patient has a one pack per day smoking history since age 17.

3. *Medications*: Fluorouracil (5-FU), Tylenol prn for back pain.

4. *Cognition/perception*: Alert and oriented x 3. Without perceptual issues at present.

5. *ROM*: WNL all extremities, trunk, and neck.

6. *Strength*: See Table 4-3. Limited strength is also complicated by significant fatigue/decreased endurance for function, especially after chemotherapy treatment.

7. *Endurance*: Resting HR = 84, BP = 138/88, RR = 20 and regular. At the end of the 6-minute walk test: HR = 120, BP = 160/94, RR = 26 with complaints of SOB.

8. *Skin/edema*: Colostomy in place with collecting bag. Otherwise without skin issues. Moderate bilateral LE edema noted. Patient does not have compression stockings at this time.

9. *Pain*: Patient has generalized complaints of stiffness secondary to immobility. Most significantly, she complains of low back pain which is a 4 on a 1 to 10 scale at rest, increasing to a 6 or 7 during transitional movements and ambulation.

10. *Neurological*: Sensation—minimal deficits in light touch and pain sensation distal LE (patient correctly identifies seven of 10 stimuli). Otherwise intact for all sensory modalities.

11. *Balance*: WNL for sitting static and dynamic balance activities. Patient requires a straight cane for short distance ambulation (ie, 20 ft for in-room function). She uses a rolling walker for support secondary to balance and endurance issues for ambulating greater distances. Protective extension and equilibrium reactions are intact.

12. *Mobility*:

Bed mobility:

- *Rolling: Independent.*
- *Bridging: Minimum assistance secondary to back pain.*
- *Supine ↔ sit: Minimum assistance secondary to back pain and decreased trunk strength.*
- *Equipment: None used presently.*

Transfers:

- *Sit → stand: Minimum assistance with straight cane or rolling walker secondary to back pain and decreased strength.*
- *Bed ↔ chair: Independent.*
- *Toilet: Supervised with a three-in-one commode over the toilet.*
- *Tub/shower: Minimum assistance with moderate cues for seat.*

<u>Table 4-3</u>

Manual Muscle Test

Left	Muscle/Muscle Group	Right	Comments
	Neck		
F+	Flexion/extension	F+	
F+	Rotation	F+	
F+	Lateral flexion	F+	
	Trunk		
P+	Flexion/extension	P+	
P+	Rotation	P+	
P+	Lateral flexion	P+	
P+	Pelvic elevation	P+	
	Upper Extremities		
WNL	Scapular abd/add	WNL	
WNL	Scapular elevation	WNL	
G-	Shoulder flexion/extension	G-	
G-	Shoulder abd/add	G-	
G-	Shoulder IR/ER	G-	
G-	Shoulder horizontal abd/add	G-	
G	Elbow flexion/extension	G	
G	Forearm pronation/supination	G	
G	Wrist flexion/extension	G	
G	MCP flexion/extension	G	
G	PIP flexion/extension	G	
G	DIP flexion/extension	G	
G	Finger abd/add	G	
G	Thumb MCP flexion/extension	G	
G	Thumb ICP flexion/extension	G	
G	Thumb abd/add	G	
G	Thumb opposition	G	
	Lower Extremities		
F+/F-	Hip flexion/extension	F+/F-	
P+/P+	Hip abd/add	P+/P+	
F/F	Hip IR/ER	F+/F+	

Left	Muscle/Muscle Group	Right	Comments
G	Knee flexion/extension	G	
F+/F+	Ankle plantar/dorsiflexion	G-/F+	
G-	Foot eversion/inversion	G-	
WNL	Great toe flexion/extension	WNL	
WNL	Toe MTP flexion/extension	WNL	
WNL	Toe IP flexion/extension	WNL	

Table 4-3 continued

abd = abduction; add = adduction; IR = internal rotation; ER = external rotation; MCP = metacarpophalangeal; PIP = proximal interphalangeal; DIP = distal interphalangeal; ICP = intermittent compression pump; WNL = within normal limits; WFL = within functional limits; G = good (80%); G+ = good (90%); F = fair (50%); F+ = fair (60%); F- = fair (40%); P = poor (20%); P+ = poor (30%); P- = poor (10%).

- *Car: Minimum assistance with minimum cues for technique.*

13. *Gait*: Patient uses a straight cane for ambulation in a room (a distance no greater than 20 ft) independently but requires supervision for any functional mobility task in a room secondary to decreased endurance and strength with patient having difficulty pacing herself. She ambulates with a forward flexed posture and a wide base of support. She uses a rolling walker for support when ambulating distances greater than 20 ft and can ambulate 75 ft x 3 during a 6-minute walk test. She requires a 60 to 90 second rest between each 75 ft distance.

14. *Stairs*: To be evaluated as patient has four steps with bilateral rails to enter her home with the bedroom on the second floor. There are full baths on the first and second floors.

15. *Functional mobility*: Patient requires supervision to minimum assistance for all functional mobility tasks at an ambulatory level.

16. *Self-care:*
- *Feeding/equipment: Independent.*
- *Bathing: Once seated on the tub seat, the patient is able to bathe herself independently with the exception of bathing her feet. She requires minimum assistance for this task as she cannot reach her feet secondary to back pain.*
- *Grooming: She is independent in grooming from a seated position at the sink and mirror.*
- *Dressing: From a seated position she is able to dress her upper body and upper trunk but requires minimum assistance for donning underwear, pants, stockings, and shoes.*

- *Toileting: She is independent in completing toilet hygiene, including colostomy care once seated on a kitchen chair in the bathroom.*
- *Fatigue and timeliness of task completion is an overriding factor affecting her function.*

17. *Home management*: Patient is now totally dependent on others to transport her children to and from activities. She continues to have housekeeping services but is no longer able to reorganize and pick up her home as she once did and cannot do the grocery shopping.

PATIENT GOALS

1. Independent self-care.
2. Independent transfers.
3. Independent functional mobility, preferable at an ambulatory level.
4. Ability to attend at least one athletic or musical event for each child weekly.
5. Return home as soon as possible.

EXERCISES FOR THE OT AND PT STUDENT

Case #19: Sonya Wellfleet

1. Using the Nagi scheme of disability, present the active pathology(ies), impairments, functional limitations, and disabilities for this case.
2. Do you think the patient's goals are realistic? Why or why not? If not, what strategies would you use to help the patient focus on more realistic goals?

3. Write an assessment and plan for the patient case(s) assigned. Include appropriate short-term and long-term goals.

4. Present a thorough plan of care for the case (ie, what specifically would you do with this patient and why?)

5. Design a treatment session lasting 30 minutes for this patient.

6. If both occupational and physical therapy were involved with this patient, what would you see as the role for each discipline to provide an appropriate, comprehensive treatment program? Consider the concepts of cotreatment and expert consultation in your answer.

7. Based upon the pathology that the patient exhibits and the individual impairments and functional limitations, do you think the patient will ever become totally "able" again? If not, which disabilities may remain?

8. What compensatory strategies might you teach the patient in this case?

9. What type(s) of DME (orthotic, prosthetic, or adaptive equipment) might you prescribe and why?

10. What would you propose as an appropriate treatment frequency and length of stay for this patient in your treatment setting? Provide the rationale for your answer.

11. What modifications would you have to make to the plan of care if you received insurance approval for only one-half of the time requested and the patient did not want to fund therapy privately?

12. Which portion(s) of the plan of care would you delegate to an assistant? Which portion(s) to an aide/tech? Provide your rationale for your answer.

13. For physical therapy students: Using the *Guidelines for Practice*, what would be your physical therapy diagnosis for this patient?

14. What environment(s) would you choose for implementing your treatment activities?

15. What activities would you use to address this patient's values?

16. Who is this patient? What roles and activities are important to her?

EXERCISES FOR THE ASSISTANT STUDENT

Case #19: Sonya Wellfleet

1. Using the Nagi scheme of disability, present the active pathology(ies), impairments, functional limitations, and disabilities for this case.

2. Design a treatment session lasting 30 minutes for this patient.

3. If both occupational and physical therapy were involved with this patient, what would you see as the role for each discipline to provide an appropriate, comprehensive treatment program? Consider the concepts of cotreatment and expert consultation in your answer.

4. Based upon the pathology that the patient exhibits and the individual impairments and functional limitations, do you think the patient will ever become totally "able" again? If not, which disabilities may remain?

5. What compensatory strategies might you teach the patient in this case?

6. What type(s) of DME (orthotic, prosthetic, or adaptive equipment) might you prescribe and why?

7. Which portion(s) of the plan of care would you delegate to an aide/tech? Provide your rationale for your answer.

8. What environment(s) would you choose for implementing your treatment activities?

9. What activities would you use to address this patient's values?

10. Who is this patient? What roles and activities are important to her?

Deconditioning with Congestive Heart Failure and Chronic Obstructive Pulmonary Disease

Mary Rosa is a 78-year-old widow who lives alone in her two-story home of 57 years. She moved into her home after she was married for 1 year. Her husband, a fisherman, had bought the house when she was pregnant with their first child. She plans to die in her home. She has so many memories, both wonderful and sad, associated with her home and its belongings. Her beloved husband has been dead for 10 years now.

Mrs. Rosa has all she can do to keep on caring for her home. She only uses the stairs once in the morning and to go to bed each evening. Her children practically forced her to have a half-bathroom added to the first floor. Also, she is unable to access the community as she was able to do just a short year ago. Her knees make ascending/descending the stairs quite a chore. She has approximately one dozen stairs from her front door to the street.

Life has blessed her with three wonderful sons. They do her grocery shopping and take her to any appointments that she may have. They wash her windows every spring and mow her lawn. She laments at how her garden has gone to seed.

Every morning she does all of her laundry by hand and makes plenty of food just in case her sons and their families might be hungry.

Overall, her health has been unremarkable. She has degenerative joint disease (DJD), which has impaired her ability to use the stairs, and her hands are slow because her knuckles are gnarled. Also, she cannot reach into her overhead shelves in the kitchen, and reaching the closet pole is a thing of the past. She had a bout

with pneumonia last year and was subsequently diagnosed with CHF and chronic obstructive pulmonary disease (COPD).

She is managing quite well. Over the last 2 weeks, she has thought she was developing the flu. She did not have her usual "get up and go" in the morning. Also, her appetite was poor and she found herself sleeping a good part of the day. After several days, her eldest son found her sleeping in the afternoon and thought she was disoriented upon waking. Alarmed, he took her to her physician who found her listless with edema of bilateral extremities (BLE). He recommended hospitalization.

At the hospital, she was diagnosed with pneumonia, dehydration, CHF, and COPD. After a 3-day stay, she was discharged to your skilled nursing unit. Mrs. Rosa clearly states her plans to return home with the support of her family. She has lost significant weight (10 pounds)—she states the food is horrible.

The results of the initial evaluation are as follows:

1. *Perception*: The patient has had one cataract removed and is waiting for the other cataract to ripen. She wears bifocals.

2. *Cognition*: Overall, she is alert and oriented x 3. Appears to experience mild confusion upon waking and later in the day.

3. *Sensation/pain*: Sensation is WFL throughout. Patient experiences pain at all end ranges in her shoulder, fingers, and knees. She would rate it as a 4 at rest and as a 7 during activity on a scale of 1 to 10. She uses Tylenol at home for pain relief.

4. *Skin/edema*: Unremarkable.

5. *Balance*: Seated, she has good static balance and can complete minimum to moderate excursions safely. Standing balance is WFL for static and minimum excursions. Balance is affected by poor endurance.

6. *Mobility:*

Bed mobility:

- *Rolling: Minimum assistance with minimum cues using the bed rails.*
- *Bridging: Minimum assistance with minimum cues using the bed rails.*
- *Supine → sit: Moderate assistance.*
- *Equipment: Half-bed rails.*

Transfers:

- *Sit → stand: Minimum assistance with minimum cues for sequencing.*
- *Bed ↔ walker: Minimum assistance with minimum cues.*
- *Chair ↔ walker: Minimum assistance with minimum cues.*
- *Toilet ↔ walker: Minimum assistance with minimum cues.*
- *Tub/shower: NT.*
- *Car: NT.*

7. *Wheelchair mobility*: Wheelchair is used only for distance with maximum assistance.

8. *Gait/functional mobility*: Rolling walker with a carrying bag for all transfers and ambulating to bathroom. Patient ambulates with slight knee flexion and a shuffling gait. Patient is fatigued after 20 ft; she requires minimum assistance with maximum cues for encouragement. She states she just wants to lie down and sleep.

9. *Self-care (right dominant)*

- *Feeding/equipment: Can independently feed herself. However, she frequently drops the utensil and prefers to use a spoon. At home, she ate more finger foods, puréed, or drank soups from a mug due to her hand functionality. Also, she states the food just doesn't taste good to her.*
- *Bathing: Sink level, seated, bathes upper body with moderate assistance secondary to decreased ROM, strength, and endurance. Bathes lower body with maximum assistance. Stand/wash presents a safety issue due to fatigue.*
- *Grooming: If given adequate time, she is able to perform all grooming. She uses BUE to comb her hair due to ROM and will use other UE as a functional assistant.*
- *Dressing: Seated in chair with armrests. She requires moderate assistance for her upper body and maximum assistance to don undergarments. Dresses lower body with maximum assistance to don clothing over feet. Stand/hike requires moderate assistance.*
- *Toileting: Assistance level varies with time of day and fatigue. She requires moderate assistance later in the day and if she has a bowel movement.*
- *Home management: Not appropriate at this time. Will be assessed at a later date.*

- *Leisure/community: Currently, listening to the radio and visiting with her family.*

10. *ROM*: See Table 5-1.

11. *Strength*: See Table 5-2.

PATIENT GOALS

1. Independent toileting.
2. Independent bed mobility.
3. Independent transfers.
4. Independent self-care.
5. Independent ambulation, hopefully without a device.
6. Independent light home management.
7. To return to home in the community.

EXERCISES FOR THE OT AND PT STUDENT

Case #20: Mary Rosa

1. Using the Nagi scheme of disability, present the active pathology(ies), impairments, functional limitations, and disabilities for this case.

2. Do you think the patient's goals are realistic? Why or why not? If not, what strategies would you use to help the patient focus on more realistic goals?

3. Write an assessment and plan for the patient case(s) assigned. Include appropriate short-term and long-term goals.

4. Present a thorough plan of care for the case (ie, what specifically would you do with this patient and why?).

5. Design a treatment session lasting 30 minutes for this patient.

6. If both occupational and physical therapy were involved with this patient, what would you see as the role for each discipline to provide an appropriate, comprehensive treatment program? Consider the concepts of cotreatment and expert consultation in your answer.

7. Based upon the pathology that the patient exhibits and the individual impairments and functional limitations, do you think the patient will ever become totally "able" again? If not, which disabilities may remain?

8. What compensatory strategies might you teach the patient in this case?

9. What type(s) of DME (orthotic, prosthetic, or adaptive equipment) might you prescribe and why?

10. What would you propose as an appropriate treatment frequency and length of stay for this patient in your treatment setting? Provide the rationale for your answer.

11. What modifications would you have to make to the plan of care if you received insurance approval for only one-half of the time requested and the patient did not want to fund therapy privately?

<u>Table 5-1</u>

Range of Motion

Left	Joint/Joint Complexes	Right	Comments
	Neck		
½ → ¾ ROM	Flexion/extension	½ → ¾ ROM	
½ → ¾ ROM	Rotation	½ → ¾ ROM	
½ → ¾ ROM	Lateral flexion	½ → ¾ ROM	
	Trunk		
WFL	Flexion/extension	WFL	
WFL	Rotation	WFL	
WFL	Lateral flexion	WFL	
WFL	Pelvic elevation	WFL	
	Upper Extremities		
WFL	Scapular abd/add	WFL	
WFL	Scapular elevation	WFL	
≈ 80/full	Shoulder flexion/extension	≈ 70/full	
≈ 80/full	Shoulder abd/add	≈ 70/full	
WFL/ ≈ 30	Shoulder IR/ER	WFL/ ≈ 25	
NT	Shoulder horizontal abd/add	NT	
WFL	Elbow flexion/extension	WFL	
WFL	Forearm pronation/supination	WFL	
≈ ¾ ROM	Wrist flexion/extension	≈ ¾ ROM	
¾ ROM	MCP flexion/extension	≈ ¾ ROM	
¾ ROM	PIP flexion/extension	≈ ¾ ROM	
¾ ROM	DIP flexion/extension	≈ ¾ ROM	
¾ ROM	Finger abd/add	≈ ¾ ROM	
¾ ROM	Thumb MCP flexion/extension	≈ ¾ ROM	
¾ ROM	Thumb ICP flexion/extension	≈ ¾ ROM	
¾ ROM	Thumb abd/add	≈ ¾ ROM	
¾ ROM	Thumb opposition	≈ ¾ ROM	
	Lower Extremities		
50	SLR	60	
¾ ROM	Hip flexion/extension	WFL/0	
¾ ROM	Hip abd/add		

<u>Table 5-1 continued</u>

Left	Joint/Joint Complexes	Right	Comments
¾ ROM	Hip IR/ER	¾ ROM	
¾ ROM	Knee flexion/extension	¾ ROM	
WFL/-10	Ankle plantar/dorsiflexion	WFL/-10	
WFL	Foot eversion/inversion	WFL	
WFL	Great toe flexion/extension	WFL	
WFL	Toe MTP flexion/extension	WFL	
WFL	Toe IP flexion/extension	WFL	

abd = abduction; add = adduction; IR = internal rotation; ER = external rotation; MCP = metacarpophalangeal; PIP = proximal interphalangeal; DIP = distal interphalangeal; ICP = intermittent compression pump; WNL = within normal limits; WFL = within functional limits; SLR = straight leg raise.

<u>Table 5-2</u>

Manual Muscle Test

Left	Muscle/Muscle Group	Right	Comments
	Neck		
F+	Flexion/extension	F+	
F+	Rotation	F+	
F+	Lateral flexion	F+	
	Trunk		
G	Flexion/extension	G	
G	Rotation	G	
G	Lateral flexion	G	
G	Pelvic elevation	G	
	Upper Extremities		
F+	Scapular abd/add	F+	
G	Scapular elevation	G	
F	Shoulder flexion/extension	F	
F	Shoulder abd/add	F	
G/F	Shoulder IR/ER	G/F	
F	Shoulder horizontal abd/add	F	
F+	Elbow flexion/extension	F+	

Table 5-2 continued

Left	Muscle/Muscle Group	Right	Comments
F+	Forearm pronation/supination	F+	
F+	Wrist flexion/extension	F+	
F	MCP flexion/extension	F	
F	PIP flexion/extension	F	
F	DIP flexion/extension	F	
F	Finger abd/add	F	
F	Thumb MCP flexion/extension	F	
F	Thumb ICP flexion/extension	F	
F	Thumb abd/add	F	
F	Thumb opposition	F	
Lower Extremities			
F/F+	Hip flexion/extension	F/F+	
F+/G	Hip abd/add	F+/G	
G/F+	Hip IR/ER	G/F+	
F	Knee flexion/extension	F	
F+/G	Ankle plantar/dorsiflexion	F+/G	
F+/G	Foot eversion/inversion	F+/G	
F+/G	Great toe flexion/extension	F+/G	
F+/G	Toe MTP flexion/extension	F+/G	
F+/G	Toe IP flexion/extension	F+/G	

abd = abduction; add = adduction; IR = internal rotation; ER = external rotation; MCP = metacarpophalangeal; PIP = proximal interphalangeal; DIP = distal interphalangeal; ICP = intermittent compression pump; WNL = within normal limits; WFL = within functional limits; G = good (80%); G+ = good (90%); F = fair (50%); F+ = fair (60%); F- = fair (40%); P = poor (20%); P+ = poor (30%); P- = poor (10%).

12. Which portion(s) of the plan of care would you delegate to an assistant? Which portion(s) to an aide/tech? Provide your rationale for your answer.

13. For physical therapy students: Using the *Guidelines for Practice*, what would be your physical therapy diagnosis for this patient?

14. What environment(s) would you choose for implementing your treatment activities?

15. What activities would you use to address this patient's values?

16. Who is this patient? What roles and activities are important to her?

EXERCISES FOR THE ASSISTANT STUDENT

Case #20: Mary Rosa

1. Using the Nagi scheme of disability, present the active pathology(ies), impairments, functional limitations, and disabilities for this case.

2. Design a treatment session lasting 30 minutes for this patient.

3. If both occupational and physical therapy were involved with this patient, what would you see as the role for each discipline to provide an appropriate, comprehensive treat-

ment program? Consider the concepts of cotreatment and expert consultation in your answer.

4. Based upon the pathology that the patient exhibits and the individual impairments and functional limitations, do you think the patient will ever become totally "able" again? If not, which disabilities may remain?

5. What compensatory strategies might you teach the patient in this case?

6. What type(s) of DME (orthotic, prosthetic, or adaptive equipment) might you prescribe and why?

7. Which portion(s) of the plan of care would you delegate to an aide/tech? Provide your rationale for your answer.

8. What environment(s) would you choose for implementing your treatment activities?

9. What activities would you use to address this patient's values?

10. Who is this patient? What roles and activities are important to her?

Left Lower Extremity Amputation with Insulin-Dependent Diabetes Mellitus and Peripheral Vascular Disease

Mary Gaines is a 65-year-old retired registered nurse who was widowed 5 years ago when her husband died suddenly of a myocardial infarction. At the time of his death, she suffered great depression, which was treated with antidepressants and counseling. She no longer requires pharmacologic management of her depression but benefits greatly from the weekly support group for widows and widowers, which she attends faithfully.

Shortly after her husband's death, she found it best to sell the home in which she and her husband had lived for 40 years. She now lives in a first-floor garden-style condominium. Prior to her current injury, she was independent in all ADL, including driving and community mobility at an ambulatory level. She does report, however, that recently she has begun to slow down, finding many tasks labor intensive and leaving her short of breath. Her favorite hobby is playing bridge with her many friends in the town bridge club. She also enjoys sewing, knitting, and playing with her two grandchildren, ages 3 and 6, who visit her often.

Six days ago, Mary dropped a glass of water on the floor and although she thought she had thoroughly cleaned up the mess, several small pieces of glass remained on the floor. The next day she cut her left foot on a broken piece of a glass while walking barefoot in her kitchen. The cut became infected and she was admitted to the hospital for IV antibiotic treatment. The infection became worse, and when gangrene began to develop, she was seen for a vascular surgery consult. Considering her 50-year history of IDDM and 10-year history of severe peripheral vascu-

lar disease, it was recommended that she have a left below knee amputation. She had this done on the 12th day of her admission and was discharged to home 4 days later, where she functions at a wheelchair level with the assistance of family, friends, and a home health aide whom she pays privately. She is referred to your outpatient rehabilitation program for further preprosthetic training and the goal of prosthetic fitting in the next 2 weeks as the healing of the residual limb allows.

She presents to you in the clinic with the following:

1. *Significant past medical history*: Mild obesity, HTN, mild angina x 10 years, peripheral vascular disease (PVD) x 10 years with a history of mild intermittent claudication when walking distances greater than one-quarter mile. She smokes one to one and one-half packs of cigarettes per day and has done so for the past 50 years.

2. *Medications*: Tenormin, nitroglycerin tabs prn, darvon for pain prn, and coumadin. NPH regular and ultralente insulin.

3. *Cognition/perception*: WNL

4. *Sensation*: Moderately impaired for light touch, pain, and temperature right distal LE (below the knee to the sole of the foot) with the ability to accurately identify five of 10 stimuli. Minimal deficits noted in these areas (seven of 10 stimuli accurately identified) left of residual limb. Patient describes some phantom sensations which are not painful at this time.

5. *ROM*: See Table 5-3.

6. *Strength*: See Table 5-4.

7. *Balance*: WNL in sitting; however, patient requires a standard walker to maintain balance once independently attained from sitting.

8. *Pain*: Patient reports mild constant pain in residual limb at rest, increasing to moderate to severe with ROM and active movement of the limb.

9. *Skin/edema*: Staples remain intact on the residual limb. The incision appears clean and dry with patient reporting only occasional episodes of minimal drainage. The residual limb is moderately edematous and is compressed with ace wraps at all times. The patient is able to remove the wrap and inspect the limb four times daily as recommended by her surgeon. She can also rewrap the limb independently.

10. *Mobility*

    - *Bed mobility: Independent bed mobility with slow, deliberate movement, especially for supine to sit and sit to supine as she guards her left leg closely so as not to hit it on any surface.*

    - *Transfers: Transfers are independent with a walker without a prosthesis for home-level function and car transfers. Awaiting prosthetic fitting to determine transfer status with her prosthesis.*

    - *Gait: Patient is able to ambulate 20 ft with a standard walker without complaints of angina or heart rate and*

<u>Table 5-3</u>
Range of Motion

Left	Joint/Joint Complexes	Right	Comments
	Neck		
WNL	Flexion/extension	WNL	
WNL	Rotation	WNL	
WNL	Lateral flexion	WNL	
	Trunk		
WNL	Flexion/extension	WNL	
WNL	Rotation	WNL	
WNL	Lateral flexion	WNL	
WNL	Pelvic elevation	WNL	
	Upper Extremities		
WNL	Scapular abd/add	WNL	
WNL	Scapular elevation	WNL	
WNL	Shoulder flexion/extension	WNL	
WNL	Shoulder abd/add	WNL	
WNL	Shoulder IR/ER	WNL	
WNL	Shoulder horizontal abd/add	WNL	
WNL	Elbow flexion/extension	WNL	
WNL	Forearm pronation/supination	WNL	
WNL	Wrist flexion/extension	WNL	
WNL	MCP flexion/extension	WNL	
WNL	PIP flexion/extension	WNL	
WNL	DIP flexion/extension	WNL	
WNL	Finger abd/add	WNL	
WNL	Thumb MCP flexion/extension	WNL	
WNL	Thumb ICP flexion/extension	WNL	
WNL	Thumb abd/add	WNL	
WNL	Thumb opposition	WNL	
	Lower Extremities		
50 degrees	SLR	68 degrees	Pain with SLR secondary to muscle tightness, arterial disease bilaterally as well as postsurgical pain on the left side

Table 5-3 continued

Left	Joint/Joint Complexes	Right	Comments
WFL	Hip flexion/extension	WFL	
WFL	Hip abd/add	WFL	
WFL	Hip IR/ER	WFL	
WFL	Knee flexion/extension	WFL	
N/A	Ankle plantar/dorsiflexion	WNL/0 degrees	
N/A	Foot eversion/inversion	Min ↓	
N/A	Great toe flexion/extension	Min ↓	
N/A	Toe MTP flexion/extension	Min ↓	
N/A	Toe IP flexion/extension	Min ↓	

Min ↓ = minimal decrease; abd = abduction; add = adduction; IR = internal rotation; ER = external rotation; MCP = metacarpophalangeal; PIP = proximal interphalangeal; DIP = distal interphalangeal; ICP = intermittent compression pump; WNL = within normal limits; WFL = within functional limits; SLR = straight leg raise.

Table 5-4

Manual Muscle Test

Left	Muscle/Muscle Group	Right	Comments
	Neck		
WFL	Flexion/extension	WFL	
WFL	Rotation	WFL	
WFL	Lateral flexion	WFL	
	Trunk		
Min ↓	Flexion/extension	Min	
Min ↓	Rotation	Min	
Min ↓	Lateral flexion	Min	
Min ↓	Pelvic elevation	Min	
	Upper Extremities		
WNL	Scapular abd/add	WNL	
WNL	Scapular elevation	WNL	
WNL	Shoulder flexion/extension	WNL	
WNL	Shoulder abd/add	WNL	
WNL	Shoulder IR/ER	WNL	

Table 5-4 continued

Left	Muscle/Muscle Group	Right	Comments
WNL	Shoulder horizontal abd/add	WNL	
WNL	Elbow flexion/extension	WNL	
WNL	Forearm pronation/supination	WNL	
WNL	Wrist flexion/extension	WNL	
WNL	MCP flexion/extension	WNL	
WNL	PIP flexion/extension	WNL	
WNL	DIP flexion/extension	WNL	
WNL	Finger abd/add	WNL	
WNL	Thumb MCP flexion/extension	WNL	
WNL	Thumb ICP flexion/extension	WNL	
WNL	Thumb abd/add	WNL	
WNL	Thumb opposition	WNL	
	Lower Extremities		
F+/F-	Hip flexion/extension	G/F+	
F+/F	Hip abd/add	G-/F+	
F+/F+	Hip IR/ER	G/G	
F+/F+	Knee flexion/extension	G/G+	Left limited by pain
N/A	Ankle plantar/dorsiflexion	G	
N/A	Foot eversion/inversion	G	
N/A	Great toe flexion/extension	G	
N/A	Toe MTP flexion/extension	G	
N/A	Toe IP flexion/extension	G	

BP rising above doctor prescribed guidelines of 130 bpm and 160/95. She has moderate complaints of pain with ambulation. She is fearful of trying to use a rolling walker to decrease the cardiac work of this task, as she states that she feels, "it will get away" from her. She is unable to ascend and descend stairs at this point.

PATIENT GOALS

1. Independent don/doff of her new prosthesis.
2. Independent ambulation with a prosthesis but without a device. Distances sufficient for performance of community mobility (ie, to go to her support group and play bridge).
3. Independent transfers with her prosthesis.
4. Return to driving.
5. Independent performance of a daily exercise routine to maximize function for the rest of her life.
6. Independent home management.

EXERCISES FOR THE OT AND PT STUDENT

Case #21: Mary Gaines

1. Using the Nagi scheme of disability, present the active pathology(ies), impairments, functional limitations, and disabilities for this case.

2. Do you think the patient's goals are realistic? Why or why not? If not, what strategies would you use to help the patient focus on more realistic goals?

3. Write an assessment and plan for the patient case(s) assigned. Include appropriate short-term and long-term goals.

4. Present a thorough plan of care for the case (ie, what specifically would you do with this patient and why?)

5. Design a treatment session lasting 30 minutes for this patient.

6. If both occupational and physical therapy were involved with this patient, what would you see as the role for each discipline to provide an appropriate, comprehensive treatment program? Consider the concepts of cotreatment and expert consultation in your answer.

7. Based upon the pathology that the patient exhibits and the individual impairments and functional limitations, do you think the patient will ever become totally "able" again? If not, which disabilities may remain?

8. What compensatory strategies might you teach the patient in this case?

9. What type(s) of DME (orthotic, prosthetic, or adaptive equipment) might you prescribe and why?

10. What would you propose as an appropriate treatment frequency and length of stay for this patient in your treatment setting? Provide the rationale for your answer.

11. What modifications would you have to make to the plan of care if you received insurance approval for only one-half of the time requested and the patient did not want to fund therapy privately?

12. Which portion(s) of the plan of care would you delegate to an assistant? Which portion(s) to an aide/tech? Provide your rationale for your answer.

13. For physical therapy students: Using the *Guidelines for Practice*, what would be your physical therapy diagnosis for this patient?

14. What environment(s) would you choose for implementing your treatment activities?

15. What activities would you use to address this patient's values?

16. Who is this patient? What roles and activities are important to her?

EXERCISES FOR THE ASSISTANT STUDENT

Case #21: Mary Gaines

1. Using the Nagi scheme of disability, present the active pathology (ies), impairments, functional limitations, and disabilities for this case.

2. Design a treatment session lasting 30 minutes for this patient.

3. If both occupational and physical therapy were involved with this patient, what would you see as the role for each discipline to provide an appropriate, comprehensive treatment program? Consider the concepts of cotreatment and expert consultation in your answer.

4. Based upon the pathology that the patient exhibits and the individual impairments and functional limitations, do you think the patient will ever become totally "able" again? If not, which disabilities may remain?

5. What compensatory strategies might you teach the patient in this case?

6. What type(s) of DME orthotic, prosthetic, or adaptive equipment) might you prescribe and why?

7. Which portion(s) of the plan of care would you delegate to an aide/tech? Provide your rationale for your answer.

8. What environment(s) would you choose for implementing your treatment activities?

9. What activities would you use to address this patient's values?

10. Who is this patient? What roles and activities are important to her?

ABBREVIATIONS

↑	increase
↓	decrease
x 1	one time, one person
2°	secondary to
a	before
abd/add	abduction/adduction
ADL	activities of daily living
AFO	ankle/foot orthosis
amb	ambulation
≈	approximate
AAROM	active assistive range of motion
AROM	active range of motion
B	bilateral
bid	twice daily
BLE	bilateral lower extremities
bpm	beats per minute
c	with
CARF	Commission on Accreditation of Rehabilitation Facilities
CHF	congestive heart failure
c/o	complains of
COPD	chronic obstructive pulmonary disease
COTA	Certified Occupational Therapy Assistant
CPM	continuous passive motion
CVA	cerebrovascular accident
d/c	discharge, discontinue
DEP	data, evaluation, performance goals
DJD	degenerative joint disease
DME	durable medical equipment
DOB	date of birth
Dx	diagnosis
ED	emergency department
ER	emergency room
ex	exercise
FES	functional electrical stimulation
FOR	functional outcome report
f/u	follow-up
G/H	glenohumeral joint
HTN	hypertension
HNP	herniated nucleosus pulposus
Hx	history
I	independently
ICP	intermittent compression pump
int	internal
JCAHO	Joint Commission on Accreditation of Healthcare Organizations
JRA	juvenile rheumatoid arthritis
KAFO	knee/ankle/foot orthosis
L	left
lat	lateral
LBP	low back pain
LLE	left lower extremity
LOB	loss of balance
LTG	long term goal
LUE	left upper extremity
mets	metastasis
min	minimum/minimal
mmHg	millimeters of mercury
MMT	manual muscle test
N/A	not applicable

neg	negative	**s/p**	status post
noc	night	**TED**	thromboembolic device
NWB	nonweightbearing	**temp**	temperature
OA	osteoarthritis	**THA**	total hip arthroplasty
OOB	out of bed	**THP**	total hip precautions
out pt	outpatient	**THR**	total hip replacement
OP	osteoporosis	**ther ex**	therapeutic exercise
OT	occupational therapist	**tid**	three times daily
p	after	**TKA**	total knee arthroplasty
per	by	**TKR**	total knee replacement
peri-area	perineal area	**TKE**	total knee extension
pm	afternoon	**TDWB**	touch down weightbearing
PRE	progressive resistive exercise	**tx**	treatment
prn	as needed	**UE**	upper extremity
PROM	passive range of motion	**w/**	with
PSP	problem, status, plan	**WBAT**	weightbearing as tolerated
PSPG	problem, status, plan, goals	**wc or w/c**	wheelchair
pt	patient	**WFL**	within functional limits
PT	physical therapist	**WNL**	within normal limits
PTA	physical therapist assistant	**w/o or s**	without
R	right	**wt**	weight
RLE	right lower extremity	**y.o.**	years old
RUE	right upper extremity		

INDEX